Gastrointestinal

Acute Abdominal Trauma in Infants And Children

Acute abdominal trauma in children may be blunt (85%) or penetrating (15%). Blunt trauma from motor vehicle accidents, pedestrian injuries (running into traffic), lap belt injury, and sports injuries are common causes of abdominal injury. About 5% of abdominal injuries are related to child abuse, such as punching or kicking a child in the abdomen.

- Blunt injuries comprise crush (compression), shear (tearing), and burst (sudden increased pressure). Because the rib cage in a young child remains elastic, there may be major internal damage from blunt trauma without rib fractures.
- Penetrating wounds, on the other hand, may be related to accidental impaling but are almost always related to gunshot wounds (high energy) or knife assaults (low energy). Gunshot wounds tend to cause more extensive damage than stab wounds. Children's organs are larger in proportion to body size than those of adults, so they are more at risk from penetrating wounds.

Splenic Injury
The spleen is the most frequently injured solid organ in blunt trauma in children because it's not well protected by the elastic rib cage and is very vascular. Symptoms may be very non-specific. Kehr sign (radiating pain in left shoulder) indicates intra-abdominal bleeding and Cullen sign (ecchymosis around umbilicus) indicates hemorrhage from ruptured spleen. Some children may have right upper abdominal pain although diffuse abdominal pain often occurs with blood loss, associated with hypotension.

Splenic injuries are classified according to the degree of injury:
1. Tear in splenic capsules or hematoma.
2. Laceration of parenchyma (<3 cm).
3. Laceration of parenchyma (>3cm).
4. Multiple lacerations of parenchyma or burst-type injury.

Treatment may be supportive if injury is not severe; otherwise, suturing of the spleen may be needed. Because children risk infection with splenectomy, every effort (bed rest, transfusion, reduced activity for at least 8 weeks) is done to avoid surgery because the spleen will often heal spontaneously.

Hepatic Injury
Hepatic injury is the most common cause of death from abdominal trauma and is often associated with multiple organ damage, so symptoms may be non-specific. Automobile accidents cause most blunt trauma but accidents with mountain bikes account for increasing hematomas of the central area of the liver. Neonatal hepatic injuries are often misdiagnosed. Elevation in liver transaminase levels indicates damage that may require CT examination with double contrast. Liver injuries are classified according to the degree of injury:

I. Tears in capsule with hematoma.
II. Laceration(s) of parenchyma (<3 cm).
III. Laceration(s) of parenchyma (<3 cm).
IV. Destruction of 25-75% of lobe from burst injury.
V. Destruction of >75% of lobe from burst injury.
VI. Avulsion [tearing away].

Almost all hepatic injuries in children (97%) are treated conservatively, primarily because studies show that most hemorrhage stops prior to surgery. Injuries may take 3-12 months to heal with supportive treatment and close monitoring.

Gastric and Intestinal Injuries
Gastric injuries in children may result in perforation, primarily at the greater curvature. The risk increases if children are injured with a full stomach after eating a meal and suffer a lap belt injury or fall over the handlebars of a bicycle. Perforation results in severe pain, rigid abdomen, and bloody nasogastric drainage with peritonitis developing within hours, so early diagnosis and surgical repair must be done. Intestinal injuries from blunt trauma are rare in children although contusions and rupture can occur from lap belt injuries. Indications of rupture often appear 24-48 hours later when the child presents with symptoms of peritonitis, such as distention, abdominal pain, absent bowel sounds, leukocytosis, fever, dyspnea, nausea and vomiting. Prompt antibiotic therapy and surgical repair with peritoneal lavage must be done. The abdominal wound may be left open to heal by secondary intention.

Pancreatic Injuries
Pancreatic injury can result from motor vehicle or handlebar accidents or assault with impact to the abdominal area although it is not a common injury. Penetrating injuries (gunshot wounds and stabbings) are more common. Because of the location of the pancreas, impact compresses it against the vertebral column. About 90% of children with pancreatic injury sustain other abdominal injuries as well, making diagnosis difficult. Symptoms may include diffuse abdominal or epigastric pain and well as vomiting of bile.

Pancreatic injuries are classified according to degree of injury:
1. Contusion, laceration but ducts intact.
2. Distal transection or injury of parenchyma with ductal injury.
3. Proximal transection or injury of parenchyma with probable ductal injury.
4. Combined injury of pancreas and duodenum.

CT scans provide the best tool for diagnosis. Surgical exploration and repair of severe damage is the most common treatment. Pancreatitis and diabetes mellitus may be long-term sequelae.

Compartment Syndrome
Abdominal trauma with pronounced shock increases risk of compartment syndrome for a number of reasons:
- Edema of the intestines because of trauma and surgical manipulation.
- Capillary leakage.
- Hemorrhage (retroperitoneal).
- Abdominal packing left in place to control bleeding.

- IV crystalloid administration.

Pressure within the abdomen may begin to rise rapidly if the abdomen is closed, resulting in decreased cardiac output from pressure on the vena cava, increased airway pressures and acute respiratory distress syndrome, decreased urinary output with decrease in renal blood flow and glomerular filtration, increased central venous pressure resulting in increased intracranial pressure and cerebral edema. *Diagnosis* is by measurement of intra-abdominal pressure (>25 cm H_2O) by Foley catheter or NG tube with pressure transducer or water-column manometry. If risk for compartment syndrome exists, the wound should not be closed. Sudden release of pressure and reperfusion may cause acidosis, vasodilation, and cardiac arrest, so the child should be given crystalloid solutions before decompression.

Peritonitis

Peritonitis (inflammation of the peritoneum) may be primary (from infection of blood or lymph) or, more commonly, secondary, related to perforation or trauma of the gastrointestinal tract, Common causes include perforated bowel, ruptured appendix, abdominal trauma, abdominal surgery, peritoneal dialysis or chemotherapy, or leakage of sterile fluids, such as blood, into the peritoneum. *Diagnosis* is made according to clinical presentation, abdominal x-rays, which may show distention of the intestines or air in the peritoneum, and laboratory findings, such as leukocytosis. Blood cultures may indicate sepsis.

Symptoms of peritonitis are those of an acute abdomen.

Symptoms	Treatment
<ul><li>Diffuse abdominal pain with rebound tenderness (Blumberg's sign).</li><li>Abdominal rigidity.</li><li>Paralytic ileus.</li><li>Fever (with infection).</li><li>Nausea and vomiting.</li><li>Sinus tachycardia.</li></ul>	<ul><li>Intravenous fluids and electrolytes.</li><li>Broad-spectrum antibiotics.</li><li>Laparoscopy as indicated to determine cause of peritonitis and effect repair.</li></ul>

Acute Gastrointestinal Bleeding

Gastrointestinal bleeding is unusual in children, but the age of the child and symptoms can indicate the area that is bleeding:

- Neonates: Apparent bleeding may occur from the infant swallowing maternal blood during delivery or from allergy to milk protein, but actual bleeding may result from mucosal erosion from increased gastric acid or from maternal medications (aspirin, phenobarbitol) that cause problems with coagulation, or medications to the infant, such as indomethacin and dexamethasone. Bleeding indicates necrotizing enterocolitis, Hirschsprung's disease, volvulus, or coagulopathies.
- Older infants: Intussusception and mucosal lesions cause most bleeding.

- Children/adolescents: Wide range of disorders may cause bleeding, including ulcers, inflammatory bowel disease, infectious diarrhea. Stress ulcers may relate to system disease.

Symptoms	Treatment
• Vomiting blood, bloody or tarry stools. • Abdominal distention. • Hypotension with tachycardia.	• Fluid replacement with transfusions is necessary. • Identification and treatment of underlying problem. • Endoscopy or push enteroscopy for upper GI bleeding. • Colonoscopy for lower GI bleeding.

Stress-Related Erosive Syndrome

Stress-related erosive syndrome (SRES) (stress ulcers) occurs most frequently in children who are critically ill, such as those with severe or multi-organ trauma, mechanical ventilation, sepsis, severe burns, and head injury with increased intracranial pressure. Stress induces changes in the gastric mucosal lining and decreased perfusion of the mucosa, causing ischemia. SRES involves hemorrhage in ≥30% with mortality rates of 30-80% so prompt identification and treatment is critical. The lesions tend to be diffuse, so they are more difficult to treat than peptic ulcers.

Symptoms	Treatment
• Coffee ground emesis. • Hematemesis. • Abdominal discomfort.	**Prophylaxis** in those at risk: • Sucralfate (Carafate®) protects mucosa against pepsin. • Famotidine (Pepcid®), nizatidine (Axid®), ranitidine (Zantac®) or cimetidine (Tagamet®) reduces gastric secretions. **Treatment for active bleeding** includes: • Intraarterial infusion of vasopressin. • Intraarterial embolization. • Oversewing of ulcers or total gastrectomy if bleeding persists.

Bowel Infarction and Perforation

Bowel infarction is ischemia of the intestines related to severely restricted blood supply. It can be the result of a number of different conditions, such as volvulus and malrotation defects, and may follow untreated bowel obstruction. Children present with acute abdomen and shock, and mortality rates are very high even with resection of infarcted bowel.

Bowel perforation occurs when the intestine erodes or is perforated and creates an opening through which fecal material and bacteria can enter the abdominal cavity. Perforation may be caused by ingestion of foreign objects, abdominal trauma, or disease, such as necrotizing enterocolitis. The perforation may be small initially, but it can enlarge to encompass a large area. Bowel perforation can occur with endoscopic examinations and surgical manipulation as well. Symptoms include abdominal pain and distention, nausea and vomiting, and fever.

Immediate surgical repair and sometimes resection of part of the bowel is necessary to prevent life-threatening peritonitis.

Bowel Obstructions

Bowel obstruction occurs when there is a mechanical obstruction of the passage of intestinal contents because of constriction of the lumen, occlusion of the lumen, or lack of muscular contractions (paralytic ileus). Obstruction may be caused by congenital or acquired abnormalities/disorders:

Small bowel obstructions	Large bowel obstructions
• Duodenal atresia • Malrotation and volvulus • Jejunoileal atresia • Meconium ileus • Meconium peritonitis	• Hirschsprung's disease • Anorectal malformations • Meconium plug syndrome
Symptoms of bowel obstructions	
Abdominal pain and distention. Abdominal rigidity. Vomiting and dehydration. Diminished or no bowel sounds. Severe constipation (obstipation). Respiratory distress from diaphragm pushing against pleural cavity. Shock as plasma volume diminishes and electrolytes enter intestines from bloodstream. Sepsis as bacteria proliferates in bowel and invade bloodstream.	

Treatment depends on cause and includes barium enema and surgical repair.

Necrotizing Enterocolitis

Necrotizing enterocolitis is an inflammatory bowel disease affecting primarily preterm/premature infants, characterized by an immature bowel that has suffered an hypoxic episode with resultant inflammation and necrosis of the intestinal wall, allowing gas into tissues of the wall, the portal venous system, and/or peritoneal cavity. It may result in infarction and/or perforation. The distal ileum and proximal colon are most-commonly affected. The cause is not clearly understood, but appears related to an ischemic episode, colonization by bacteria, and excess/rapid enteral feedings. Mortality rates are about 30%.

Symptoms	Treatment
• Gastric retention/ abdominal distention, vomiting (bilious). • Periods of apnea. • Occult or frank blood (25%) in stool. • Pneumatosis intestinalis (gas in intestinal wall) (75%). • Portal venous gas (10-30%). • Decrease in urinary output. • Jaundice. • Unstable temperature.	• Cessation of oral feeding and NG decompression. • Systemic antibiotics. • Correcting fluid and electrolyte imbalance. • Surgical repair with bowel resection if necessary.

Complications include short gut syndrome, strictures, impaired nutrition, delayed growth, and cholestasis.

Mesenteric Ischemia

Mesenteric ischemia occurs when intestinal circulation decreases because of thrombus formation (arterial or venous), arterial embolus, or systemic shock or drugs (such as cocaine, digoxin, and α-adrenergic agonists) resulting in intestinal vasoconstriction. Mesenteric ischemia is most common in the elderly but can occur in children. Mortality rates are very high if diagnosis and treatment is delayed for >12 hours or after onset of peritonitis. Abdominal examination may be fairly normal initially, except for pain, but progresses to indications of peritonitis and shock, with fever, pain, and abdominal distention.

Symptoms (vary)	Treatment (cause-dependent)
• Pain: Severe with sudden onset (embolism) or increasing in intensity with history of pain after meals, not usually localized. • Nausea, vomiting, and diarrhea. • Melena, hematochezia, occult blood. • Pneumatosis intestinalis (gas in intestinal wall) on radiograph.	• IV fluids. • Intubation with ventilation if necessary. • Broad-spectrum antibiotics. • Analgesics (Opioids). • Thrombolytics (tPA). • Papaverine infusion (if non-occlusive). • Anticoagulants (Heparin and/or warfarin). • Surgical repair.

Adhesions

Adhesions are fibrous bands that cause intestinal loops to adhere to areas within the abdomen that heal slowly or scar after surgery. These bands can loop around the intestines and cause them to kink or bind them to other internal organs, sometimes resulting in partial or complete intestinal obstruction. Adhesions can occur in children who have had abdominal surgery or abdominal radiation treatments or may be congenital. Adhesions may increase in size over time and become more constrictive. Long-term sequelae include infertility in adulthood (females). Symptoms, usually general abdominal discomfort, may be minimal unless obstruction occurs, at which time pain and distention becomes acute. Diagnosis is often made through exploratory surgery, as adhesions are not evident on x-ray or ultrasound. Partial obstructions may be treated with dietary modifications (liquid/low residue), although severe or complete obstructions require surgical repair.

Gastroesophageal Reflux

Gastroesophageal reflux (GER) is involuntary regurgitation of stomach contents into the esophagus, usually caused by decreased tone in the lower esophageal sphincter in children.

Symptoms	Treatment
• **Infants**: Frequent regurgitation, especially after feeding, usually not associated with respiratory distress although some children may have colicky symptoms. • **Toddler/older children:** Less obvious regurgitation because they are upright more and eat solid foods, but they may refuse food or indicate or complain of pain in epigastric region. They may exhibit failure to thrive or weight loss, asthma, cough, or pneumonia from aspiration of gastric fluids.	• **Regulating feeding:** Avoiding over-feeding and (for older children) avoiding large meals or after dinner snacking. • **Positioning:** Prone positioning after feeding/eating reduces regurgitation (although some concern remains about SIDS with infants). Placing infant in an upright position (avoiding slumping) after meals or carrying the infant upright can help. • **Medications:** Histamine-2 receptor blockers and/or antacids (without aluminum).

Omphalocele

Omphalocele is a congenital herniation of intestines or other organs through the base of the umbilicus with a protecting amniotic membrane but no skin. The sac may contain only a loop or most of bowel and the internal abdominal organs. This sac differentiates gastroschisis from omphalocele. *Diagnosis* is usually with fetal ultrasound. *Symptoms* vary widely. Maintaining integrity of tissues by keeping exposed sac or viscera moist and providing intravenous fluids is important. Small omphaloceles are repaired immediately, but more extensive repair is usually delayed until infant is stable if sac is intact. Silvadene® cream toughens the sac, which is usually covered with a silastic (plastic) pouch to protect the tissue. The abdomen may be unusually small, making correction difficult, so surgeons may wait 6-12 months while the abdominal cavity grows. Surgical repair may be done in stages over 8-10 days.

Gastroschisis

Gastroschisis is extrusion of the non-rotated midgut through the abdominal wall to the right of the umbilicus with no protective membrane covering matted, thickened loops of intestine. The abnormality is usually small, but the stomach and almost all of the small and large intestines can protrude. Because the intestines float without protection in amniotic fluid, there may be severe damage to the intestines with bowel atresia and ischemia. Gastroschisis is usually diagnosed with fetal ultrasound and is obvious at birth. These infants lose body temperature, fluids, and electrolytes and receive intravenous fluids. The exposed organs are covered with sterile plastic film for protection and to prevent fluid loss, and a naso-gastric feeding tube is inserted. Primary closure is done when infant stabilizes for small abnormalities. Larger abnormalities may require staged surgeries with only part of organs returned to cavity and the remaining covered with a Silastic pouch until the abdominal cavity grows and surgical repair can be completed.

Malrotation/Volvulus

Malrotation is a congenital defect in which the intestines are attached to the back of the abdominal wall by one single attachment rather than a broad band of attachments across the abdomen, essentially suspending the bowels so that they can easily twist, resulting in a **volvulus** (twisted bowel), cutting off blood supply. The volvulus may untwist but can lead to bowel infraction. Some children with malrotation have no symptoms, but most develop symptoms by 1 year:

Symptoms	Treatment
• Cycles of cramping pain about every 15-30 minutes that cause the child to cry and pull knees to chest. • Distended painful abdomen. • Diarrhea, bloody stools, or no stools. • Vomiting (occurring soon after crying begins usually indicates small intestine obstruction; later vomiting usually indicated large intestine blockage) • Tachycardia and tachypnea. • Decreased urinary output. • Fever.	• Surgical repair (Ladd procedure) is indicated immediately if there is volvulus, and most malrotations require surgical repair even with less severe symptoms.

Hirschsprung Disease

Hirschsprung disease (congenital aganglionic megacolon) is failure of ganglion nerve cells to migrate to part of the bowel (usually the distal colon), so that part of the bowel lacks enervation and peristalsis, causing stool to accumulate and leading to distention and megacolon. There is a genetic predisposition to the disease that affects more males than females and is associated with trisomy 21 (Down syndrome). *Symptoms* include:

Neonatal diagnosis	Infancy diagnosis	Childhood diagnosis
• Failure to pass meconium in 24-48 hours. • Poor feeding. • Bilious vomitus. • Abdominal distention.	• Chronic constipation. • Failure to thrive. • Periods of diarrhea and vomiting. • Loud gurgling bowel sounds • (With infection) Severe enterocolitis with watery diarrhea, fever, hypotension.	• Chronic constipation with ribbon-like stools. • Abdominal distention with visible peristalsis and palpable fecal abdominal mass. • Poorly-nourished. • Anemia.

Treatment includes:
Resection of aganglionic section and colorectal anastomosis. There are a number of procedures (Swenson, Duhamel, and Soave) but recently laparoscopic or trans-anal minimally-invasive approaches have proven successful.

Intussusception

Intussusception is a telescoping of one portion of the intestine into another, usually at the ileocecal valve, causing an obstruction. As the walls of the intestine come in contact, inflammation and edema cause decreased perfusion, which can result in infarction with peritonitis and death. Fecal material cannot move past the obstruction. It is most common between 3-12 months but can occur until 6 years and may relate to viral infections.

Symptoms	Treatment
• "Current jelly stool" composed of blood and mucous (occurs with 60%). • Sudden an acute episode of severe abdominal pain during which child pulls knees to chest. • Vomiting. • Lethargy and weakness. • Distended abdomen, painful to palpation. • Sausage-shaped mass in RUQ of abdomen. • Progressive fever and prostration if peritonitis occurs.	• Barium or air enema to diagnose and apply pressure that may resolve the intussusception. • Surgical repair if there is shock, peritonitis, intestinal perforation, or failure to resolve with barium/air enema

Gastrointestinal Surgical Procedures

<u>Fundoplication</u>
Fundoplication in which part of the fundus of the stomach (the upper portion) is wrapped either completely or partially around the distal esophagus and then sutured is the 3rd most common surgery for children, it is done in order to prevent regurgitation and strengthen the lower esophageal sphincter. When the stomach contracts, this shuts the sphincter, preventing backflow of gastric contents into the esophagus. This procedure is done for children with congenital abnormalities of the esophagus and for those with gastroesophageal reflux if they do not respond to medical treatment. It is also a common repair after infants have had gastrostomy tubes inserted, damaging the sphincter. There are a number of different procedures, but all are basically variations of the Nissen procedure, which involves a full 360° wrap of the esophagus. In recent years, most procedures have been done with laparoscopy, allowing for small abdominal incisions and less recovery time.

<u>Hernia Repair</u>
Hernia repair (herniorrhaphy) is the most common surgery for infants and children and is done to repair herniation of the peritoneum and a segment of bowel through the abdominal wall. Surgery is necessary to prevent an incarcerated hernia, in which the bowel twists and blood supply is compromised.

There are 3 main types:
- Inguinal: Herniation in the inguinal canal. This is common in premature or low birth-weight infants, usually males, and may occur bilaterally.

- Femoral: Herniation posterior to the inguinal ligament. This is more common in females.
- Umbilical: Herniation in the umbilical ring.

Inguinal and femoral hernias are usually repaired as soon as possible because of the danger of incarceration; however, umbilical hernias pose less concern and often heal over time without surgical repair, so it is rarely done prior to school age. If incarceration has occurred prior to surgery, the affected segment of bowel is resected. Surgery may be done laparoscopically.

Esophagogastroduodenoscopy

Esophagogastroduodenoscopy (EGD) with a flexible fiberscope equipped with a lighted fiberoptic lens allows direct inspection of the mucosa of the esophagus, stomach, and duodenum. The scope has a still or video camera attached to a monitor for viewing during the procedure. The scope may be used for biopsies or therapeutically to dilate strictures or treat gastric or esophageal bleeding. The child is positioned on the left side (head supported) to allow saliva drainage. Conscious sedation (midazolam, propofol) is commonly used along with a topical anesthetic spray or gargle to facilitate placing the lubricated tube through the mouth into the esophagus. Atropine reduces secretions. A bite guard in the mouth prevents the older children from biting the scope. The airway must be carefully monitored through the procedure (which usually takes about 30 minutes), including oximeter to measure oxygen saturation. While perforation, bleeding, or infection may occur, most complications are cardiopulmonary in nature and relate to drugs (conscious sedation) used during the procedure, so reversal agents (flumazenil, naloxone) should be available.

Hepatic Cirrhosis

Compensated, Diagnostic Procedures
Cirrhosis is a chronic hepatic disease in which normal liver tissue is replaced the fibrotic tissue that impairs liver function. There are 2 types common to children:
- Postnecrotic with broad bands of fibrotic tissue is the result of acute viral hepatitis.
- Biliary, the least common type is caused by chronic biliary obstruction (bilary atresia) and cholangitis, with resulting fibrotic tissue about the bile ducts.

Cirrhosis may result from liver damage related to chronic diseases, such as cystic fibrosis and hemophilia. Compensated cirrhosis usually involves non-specific symptoms, such as intermittent fever, epistaxis, ankle edema, indigestion, abdominal pain, and palmar erythema. Hepatomegaly and splenomegaly may also be present. Decompensated cirrhosis symptoms are more severe. Diagnosis is by history, physical examination (evidence of hepatosplenomegaly), liver function tests, abdominal ultrasound (to confirm ascites), and liver biopsy. Liver biopsy may cause bleeding, so post-procedural monitoring of hematocrit and vital signs is critical.

<u>Decompensated</u>
Decompensated cirrhosis occurs when the liver can no longer adequately synthesize proteins, clotting factors, and other substances so that portal hypertension occurs.

Symptoms	Treatment
Hepatomegaly/splenomegaly. Chronic elevated temperature. Clubbing of fingers. Purpura resulting from thrombocytopenia, with bruising and epistaxis. Portal obstruction resulting in jaundice and ascites. Bacterial peritonitis with ascites. Esophageal varices. Edema of extremities and presacral area resulting from reduced albumin in the plasma. Vitamin deficiency from interference with formation, use, and storage of vitamins, such as A, C, and K. Anemia from chronic gastritis and ↓dietary intake. Hepatic encephalopathy with alterations in mentation. Hypotension. Atrophy of gonads.	Treatment varies according to the symptoms and is supportive rather than curative as the fibrotic changes in the liver cannot be reversed: Dietary supplements and vitamins Diuretics (potassium sparing), such as Aldactone® and Dyrenium®, to decrease ascites. Colchicine to reduce fibrotic changes. Liver transplant (the definitive treatment).

Portal Hypertension

Portal hypertension, obstructed blood flow increasing blood pressure throughout the portal venous system, prevents the liver from filtering blood and causes the development of collateral blood vessels that return unfiltered blood to the systemic circulation. Increasing serum aldosterone levels cause sodium and fluid retention in the kidneys, resulting in hypervolemia, ascites and esophageal varices. Portal hypertension can be caused by any liver disease, especially cirrhosis and inherited or acquired coagulopathies that cause thrombosis of the portal vein. Half the cases in infants and children result from intra-abdominal infections, such as neonatal sepsis or appendicitis.

Symptoms	Treatment
• Ascites with distended abdomen. • Esophageal varices with bleeding. • Dyspnea. • Abdominal discomfort. • Fluid & electrolyte imbalances.	• Restricted sodium intake. • Diuretics. • Intravenous fluid and replacement blood products. • Nutritional support (NG feedings or TPN). • Balloon tamponade and vasopressin for bleeding varices. • Endoscopic treatment of obstruction. • Portal vein shunting redirecting blood from the portal vein to the vena cava. • Liver transplant in severe cases.

Biliary Atresia

Biliary atresia is atresia (absence or closure) of bile ducts outside the liver, related to congenital abnormality, an autoimmune reaction, or viral process. Biliary atresia is progressive with inflammation causing further scarring and obstruction of bile ducts inside the liver. The bile retained in the liver causes distention and scarring. The pathologic process may begin in the fetus or shortly after birth. Surgical repair must be done within the first 2-3 months after birth to prevent irreversible damage to the liver.

Symptoms	Treatment
• Jaundice (2-3 weeks after birth). • Hepatomegaly with abdominal distention. • Light-colored stools and dark urine. • Failure to thrive related to poor metabolism of fat. • Irritability. • Splenomegaly (late sign).	• Kasai (roux-en-Y-hepatoportojejunostomy) surgical procedure removes exterior ducts transects the small intestine and connects the distal segment directly to the liver to provide bile drainage. The proximal segment is attached to the distal segment, below the liver-intestine anastomosis. • Liver transplant is required in about 20% of children

Esophageal Varices

Esophageal varices are torturous dilated veins in the submucosa of the esophagus (usually the distal portion), a complication of cirrhosis of the liver in which obstruction of the portal vein causes an increase in collateral vessels, a decrease in circulation to the liver, and an increase in pressure in the collateral vessels in the submucosa of the esophagus and stomach. This causes the vessels to dilate. Because they tend to be fragile and inelastic, they tear easily, causing sudden massive esophageal hemorrhage. Bleeding from varices occurs in 19-50% with associated mortality rates of 40-70%.

Treatment may include:

- Fluid and blood replacement.
- Intravenous vasopressin, somatostatin, and octreotide to ↓portal venous pressure and provide vasoconstriction.
- Endoscopic injection with sclerosing agents.
- Endoscopic variceal band ligation.
- Esophagogastric balloon tamponade to apply direct pressure.

Transjugular intrahepatic portosystemic shunting (TIPS) creates a channel between systemic and portal venous systems to reduce portal hypertension. A variety of other shunts may be done surgically if bleeding persists.

Malabsorption

Short Gut/Bowel Syndrome

Short gut (bowel) syndrome occurs when removal of part of the small intestine results in a malabsorptive condition. *Symptoms* relate to the amount of bowel removed and the area of resection:

- Resection of the terminal ileum interferes with absorption of bile salts and vitamin B12. If <100 cm removed, malabsorption of bile salts causes watery diarrhea. Treatment includes salt binding resins (cholestyramine 2 to 4 g three times daily). If >100 cm removed, steatorrhea with resultant malabsorption of fat-soluble vitamins occurs. Additional treatment includes low fat diet, vitamins, and calcium supplements to prevent oxalate kidney stone.
- Resection of >40-50% of small bowel results in weight loss, diarrhea, and electrolyte imbalance. If colon and 100cm of proximal jejunum are retained, a lowfat, high complex carbohydrate diet, and electrolytes may maintain nutrition, but if the colon is removed, 200 cm of jejunum is required for adequate nutrition. Otherwise, parenteral nutrition is required, and this can lead to liver failure and death or liver/intestine transplantation

Crohn's Disease

Crohn's disease manifests with inflammation of the GI system. Inflammation is transmural (often leading to intestinal stenosis and fistulas), focal and discontinuous with aphthous ulcerations progressing to linear and irregular shaped ulcerations. Granulomas may be present. Common sites of inflammation are the terminal ileum and cecum. Condition is usually chronic, but an acute flare-up may mimic appendicitis. Children may have delayed development and stunted growth, affecting adult stature. There is a genetic component to the disease.

Symptoms	Treatment
Perirectal abscess/fistula in advanced disease. Diarrhea usually present with colonic disease. May have nocturnal bowel movements, watery stools, and rectal hemorrhage. Anemia may develop with chronic bleeding. Abdominal pain most common in lower right quadrant, usually indicating transmural inflammation; may include post-prandial pain and cramping. Nausea and vomiting (usually related to strictures of small intestine). Malabsorption. Fever, night sweats.	Corticosteroids & antibiotics for acute exacerbations. Immunomodulatory agents (ciclosporine, methotrexate, azathioprine). Antidiarrheals. Aminosalicylates (Sufasalazine). Antibiotics (Ciprofloxacin, metronidazole). Tumor necrosis factor antagonists (Infliximab). Enteral feedings or TPN.

Celiac Disease, Lactose Intolerance, Parasitic Diseases

Disorder	Pathology	Symptoms	Treatment
Celiac disease	Autoimmune disorder with intolerance to gluten, which causes destruction of surface epithelium of the small intestine.	Loss of weight. Diarrhea, bloating, steatorrhea (fatty stools), azotorrhea (nitrogenous wastes in stool-urine). Anemia. Vitamin-Iron deficiency (folate, B12.	Gluten-free diet.
Lactose intolerance	Deficiency of intestina lactase causes increased lactose in intestine.	Diarrhea, cramping.	Oral lactase (Lactaid®). Dairy-free diet.
Parasitic diseases (Giardiasis, strongy-loidiasis, coccidiosis)	Parasites live-multiply within the intestines, causing damage to the intestinal mucosa.	(Varies with parasitic agent). Loss of weight. Diarrhea, steatorrhea.	Antiparasitic drugs as indicated for the specific parasite.

Gastrointestinal Feeding Tube Placement

Surgical placement: There are both open and laparoscopic surgical techniques for tubes to the stomach or jejunum. The three most common methods are the Janeway, the Stamm, and the Witzel techniques.

Endoscopic placement: Percutaneous endoscopic gastrostomy (PEG) involves intubation of the esophagus with the endoscope and insertion of a sheathed needle with a guidewire through the abdomen and stomach wall so that a catheter can be fed down the esophagus, snared, and pulled out through the opening where the needle was inserted and secured. Similar endoscopic procedures can be done in the jejunum.

Radiologic placement: Through fluoroscopy, ultrasound and/or CT, gastrostomy tube is inserted through the epigastrium and secured with a balloon and external bumper or disk. Insertion into the jejunum is done in a similar manner through the duodenum into the jejunum. A gastrojejunostomy tube, which both drains the stomach and feeds the jejunum, is another procedure.

Enteral Feedings

Nutritional Assessment
Caloric and nutritional needs for enteral feedings are assessed according to the age of the child, size, and stress factors. Breast milk is the optimal nutrition for infants. Feedings may be adjusted because of needs associated with diseases; for example, children with HF may

require fluid restriction. Formula usually contains 24/30 calories per ounce. Caloric requirements are based on the RDA and resting energy expenditure (REE), the calories needed for a child at rest:

Age	RDA: Kcal/kg/d	REE: Kcal/kg/d	Protein: g/kg/d
6 months to 1 year	90 to 108	55	2 to 2.5
1 to 3 years	85 to 102	50 to 57	1.2 to 3
4 to 6 years	70 to 90	45 to 48	1.1 to 3
7 to 10 years	60 to 70	40	1.0 to 3
11 to 13 years	45 to 55	28 to 32	1.0 to 2.5
15 to 18 years	36 to 45	25 to 27	0.8 to 1.2

Total energy expenditure (TEE) is calculated by multiplying the REE by stress factors:

Maintenance: 0.2

Activity: 0.1 to 0.25

Fever: 0.13 per degree>38°C

Burns: 0.5 to 1

Simple trauma: 0.2

Sepsis/major trauma: 0.4 to 1.5

Ventilation/sedation: 1.2 to 1.3   Growth: 0.5

Displacement of Enteral Feeding Tubes

The displacement of an enteral feeding tube is usually the result of inadequate stabilization. Foley catheters must be marked where they exit the stoma to check for migration. Gastrostomy tubes with an internal balloon or mushroom tip, measured markings, and an external disk are easier to stabilize, but internal device should be checked daily by gently pulling until resistance is felt. External stabilizing devices can be applied to the skin to hold the tube in place. The tube may also be taped to the abdomen or secured with a binder. Sometimes surgeons suture the tube in place, especially those with no balloon, such as jejunostomy tubes, which can become easily dislodged. A solid skin barrier with the tube fed through an anchored baby nipple is an inexpensive stabilizer. Position and length of tube should be carefully documented. Balloon volume should be checked weekly to insure there are no leaks. Skin beneath disks/ bumpers should be checked frequently.

Occlusion Of Enteral Feeding Tubes

Prevention of occlusion of enteral feeding tubes involves proper administration of medications and feedings, and maintaining a regular schedule of flushing. Tubes should be flushed with 5 to 30 ml of water (depending on age and size of child) at least every 4 hours as well as before and after feedings and administration of medications.

Medications should be in liquid form or crushed completely and enteric-coated or delayed release preparations should be avoided. Feeding solutions should be liquid consistency. Child should be positioned with head elevated for feedings.

Flushing of occluded tube involves first checking for kinks or obvious problems, attaching a 20-30 ml syringe and aspirating fluid. Then, 5-10 ml of water or carbonated beverage (ginger ale, cola) can be slowly instilled (over about a minute) and aspirated a number of times to try to loosen occlusion. After clamping for 10-15 minutes, the flushing procedure can be repeated with warm water/carbonated beverage. If the water or carbonated beverage fails, a multi-enzyme cocktail or pancrease and sodium bicarbonate solution succeed. If all flushing fails, the physician should be notified.

Complications of Enteral Feedings
Vomiting and/or aspiration - Causes - Tube incorrectly placed.
Delayed gastric emptying. Contaminated formula. Increased residual volume.
Solutions - Check tube position. Delay feeding one hour and check residual volume before resuming. Elevate head of bed 30-45°or have child sit in chair. Refrigerate formula, check dates and discard after 24 hours.

Diarrhea - Causes - Rapid feeding. Medications (such as antibiotics).
Solutions - Contaminated formula. Lactose intolerance. Low-fiber/hypertonic formula. Distal movement of tube.
Slow rate of feeding or use continuous drip. Evaluate medications.
Change tubing every 24 hours and avoid hanging feedings for more than 4 hours. Change formula (add fiber, decrease sodium).
Check position of tube before feedings.

Constipation - Causes Inadequate fluids. Fecal impaction. Medications. Formula.
Solutions - Increase fluids, according to age/size. Manual examination for fecal impaction. Evaluate medications. Consult dietician regarding formula.
Dehydration – Causes- Diarrhea/vomiting High protein formula. Poor fluid intake. Hyperosmotic diuresis.
Treat as for diarrhea/vomiting (above). Consult dietician for change in formula.
Solutions - Increase fluids. Monitor blood glucose levels.

Total Parenteral Nutrition

Total parenteral nutrition (TPN) is an intravenous hypertonic solution containing glucose, fat emulsion, protein, minerals, and vitamins. Long PICCs may be inserted in the basilic or cephalic veins and advanced into central circulation for short-term TPN. Central venous catheters are usually inserted into the subclavian or jugular vein and advanced to the tip of the superior vena cava for long-term TPN. Central solutions are more hypertonic than peripheral.

Precautions:
- Use aseptic technique for feedings, dressing changes.
- Use micropore filter (solutions without fat emulsion).
- Use 1.2-micron filter (solutions with fat emulsion).
- Change filters and IV tubing every 24 hours.

- Monitor VS every 4 hours.
- Check daily weight.
- Laboratory tests daily initially, 3 x weekly until stable, and then weekly: Glucose, electrolytes, CBC, urea nitrogen, and hepatic enzymes.
- Triglyceride level every 4 hours after intralipid (fats and EFAs) infusion begun to ensure level is ≤200 mg/dL.
- Check label and ingredients before administration.
- Discard cloudy solutions (contamination).
- Change solution at 24 hours.
- Check for infection

Initiating TPN

Commercially-prepared TPN solutions contain dextrose and protein (amino acids), but electrolytes, vitamins, and trace elements are individualized. A total nutrient admixture that contains fat emulsion, dextrose, and amino acids is widely used although fat emulsion may be administered separately. Peripheral TPN for children allows a dextrose solution of ≤12.5% while central TPN allows dextrose solution of ≥15%. Intralipid (fats and essential fatty acids) solutions are commercially available in 10% and 20% concentrations with 20% preferred for children (2 kcal/mL). Protein levels of 1.5 to 2 g/kg/ per day are common. Vitamins and trace minerals are usually added to meet MDRs. TPN is initiated slowly with infusion rate gradually increasing over 24 to 48 hours. Because hyperglycemia is a common complication, blood glucose levels should be monitored every 4 to 6 hours at bedside. Insulin may be ordered (sliding scale) to maintain glucose level <150 mg/dL. Infusion rate should not be changed to manage hyperglycemia or hypoglycemia. TPN should be administered with an infusion pump so that rate of infusion can be precisely managed, and the rate of infusion and amount infused should be checked every 30 to 60 minutes.

Complications -Insertion Trauma, Thrombus, Phlebitis, Fluid Imbalance

TPN complication	Signs/Symptoms	Management
Insertion trauma	Pneumothorax, hemothorax: Dyspnea, diminished breath sounds, Dysrhythmia Air embolism Brachial plexus injury: Numbness/weakness in arm	Emergency treatment as indicated, including removal/replacement of catheter.
Thrombus	Intraluminal blood clot. Occluded catheter.	Heparinization of PN solution
Phlebitis	Inflammation at insertion site (erythema, pain, edema) from infiltration into tissues.	Infusion of Intralipid solution.
Fluid Imbalance	Overload or dehydration: Change in urinary output, increase or decrease of BUN, creatinine, hematocrit, serum sodium and serum osmolality	Recalculate fluid requirements. Evaluate for fluid loss, fever, renal insufficiency, cardiac insufficiency.

Complications - Hyperglycemia, Hypoglycemia, Electrolyte Imbalance

TPN complication	Signs/Symptoms	Management
Hyperglycemia	Increase in serum glucose/urine glucose. Increased urinary output.	Decrease glucose concentration. Slow rate of infusion. Administer insulin.
Hypoglycemia	Decrease in serum glucose. Diaphore-sis, pallor. Lethargy confusion. Weak-ness, dizziness.	Stop insulin. Increase dextrose concentration. Slow rate of nfusion. Evaluate for sepsis.
Electrolyte imbalance	Varies according to imbalance. Maintenance requirements: • Na: 2 to 4 mEq/kg/d. • K: 2 to 4 mEq/kg/d. • Mg: 0.25 to 1.0 mEq/kg/d. • Ca: 0.5 to 3 mEq/kg/d. • P: 0.5 to 2 mmol/kg/d.	Frequent laboratory monitoring and adjustment in electrolyte administration

Complications - Hyperammonemia, Azotemia, Deficiency Of Efas, And Hyperlipidemia

TPN complication	Signs/Symptoms	Management
Hyper-ammonemia	Lethargy, change in mental status. Asterixis (flapping, tremors of hands).	Evaluate for hepatic insuf-ficiency. Decrease protein concentration in PN formula.
Azotemia	Evidence of dehydration: Dry mucous membranes, decreased skin turgor Increased BUN and urinary specific gravity.	Decrease amino acids in PN formula or change to NephrAmine
Deficiency of EFAs	Dry skin, flakiness. Thrombocytopenia.	Increase lipid intake with lipids at least 2 x weekly as well as oral fats (if possible) and topical fats.
Hyper-lipidemia	Triglyceride level increasing. Blood specimen cloudy.	Decrease lipid adminis-tration or stop if trigly-ceride ≥400 mg/dL. Monitor triglycerides every 4 hours initially & then daily.

Drain Types

Simple drains are latex or vinyl tubes of varying sizes and lengths inserted into a wound to provide drainage of serous material, blood, pus, or other discharge. This type of drain is usually placed through a stab wound near the area of involvement.

Penrose drains are soft rubber/latex tubes that are flat in appearance and are placed in surgical wounds to drain fluid by gravity and capillary action. They are available in various diameters and lengths.

Sump drains are double-lumen or tri-lumen tubes (with a third lumen for infusions). A large outflow lumen and small inflow lumen produces venting when air enters the inflow lumen and forces drainage into the large lumen.

Percutaneous drainage catheter is inserted into wound to provide continuous drainage for infection or symptoms from collection of drainage in the wound. Irrigation of the catheter may need to be done to maintain patency. Skin barriers and pouching systems may be necessary.

Closed Drainage Systems

Closed drainage systems use low-pressure suction to provide continuous gravity drainage of wounds. Drains are attached to collapsible suction reservoirs that provide negative pressure.

Management includes daily dressing changes about tube insertion site, inspection of skin for inflammation or drainage, monitoring type and amount of drainage from drain, and emptying device by holding it lower than the wound, opening the plug, draining, squeezing all air out to reestablish suction and negative pressure, and reinserting plug.

There are two closed drainage systems that are in frequent use:
- Jackson-Pratt® is a bulb-type drain that is about the size of a lemon. A thin plastic drain from the wound extends to a squeeze bulb that can hold about 100ml of drainage.
- Hemovac® is a round drain with coiled springs inside that are compressed after emptying to create suction. The device can hold up to 500 ml of drainage.

Liver Function Studies

Bilirubin and PT

Liver function studies	
Bilirubin	Determines the ability of the liver to conjugate and excrete bilirubin. • Direct total: 0.0-0.3 to 1.2 mg/dL • Unconjugated <1.1 mg/dL • Conjugated: < 0.3 mg/dL. • Delta: <0.2 mg/dL.
Prothrombin time (PT)	100% or clot detection in 10-13 seconds. PT increases with liver disease. Critical value: PT > 20 seconds if not receiving anticoagulation and 3 times normal control value if receiving anticoagulation. **International normalized ratio (INR)** (PT result/normal average): <2 for those not receiving anticoagulation and 2.0 to 3.0 those receiving anticoagulation. Critical value: >3 in patients receiving anticoagulation therapy.

<u>Alkaline Phosphatase, AST, ALT, GGT</u>

Alkaline phosphatase   (Normal values vary with method.)

- 1 to 5 years: Male 56 to 350 U/L, Female 73 to 378 U/L.
- 6 to 7 years: Male 70 to 364 U/L, Female 73 to 378 U/L.
- 8 years: Male 70 to 364 U/L, Female 98 to 448 U/L.
- 9 to 12 years: Male 112 to 476, Female 98 to 448 U/L.
- 13 years: Male 112 to 476 U/L, Female 56 to 350 U/L.
- 14 years: Male 112 to 476 U/L, Female 56 to 266 U/L.
- 15 years: Male 70 to 378 U/L, Female 42 to 168 U/L.
- 16 years: Male 70 to 378 U/L, Female 28 to 126 U/L.
- 17 years: Male 56 to 238 U/L, Female 28 to 126 U/L.
- I8 years; Male 56 to 182 U/L, Female 28 to 126 U/L

Increase indicates biliary tract obstruction if no bone disease.

AST (SGOT)

- 10 days to 24 months: 9 to 80 U/L.
- 2 to 29 years: Male 14 to 40 U/L, Female 13 to 35 U/L.

Increased in liver cell damage.

ALT (SGPT)

- 0 to 1 year: 13 to 45 U/L.

- 2 years to adult: Male 10 to 40 U/L, Female 7 to 35 U/L.

Increase in liver cell damage.

GGT, SGGT

Male 1 to 94 UL, Female 1 to 70 U/L.
Increase with liver disease.

LDH, NH₃, Cholesterol

Liver function studies	
LDH	<ul><li>0 to 2 years: 125 to 275 U/L.</li><li>2 to 3 years: 166 to 232 U/L.</li><li>4 to 6 years: 104 to 206 U/L.</li><li>7 to 12 years: 90 to 203 U/L.</li><li>13 to 14 years: 90 to 199 U/L.</li><li>15 to 43 years: 90 to 156 U/L.</li><li>Increase with liver disease.</li></ul>
Serum ammonia (NH₃)	<ul><li>Newborn: 90 to 150 µg/dL.</li><li>Adult male: 27 to 102 µg/dL.</li><li>Adult female: 19 to 87 µg/dL.</li><li>Increase with liver failure, GI hemorrhage, TPN.</li></ul>
Cholesterol, total HDL, LDL, Triglycerides	**Total:** <200 mg/dL. Increase with bile duct obstruction and decrease with parenchymal disease. **HDL:** >60 mg/dL. **LDL:** <100 mg/dL. **Triglycerides:**<ul><li>0 to 9 years: Male 30 to 100 mg/dL, Female 35 to 110 mg/dL</li><li>10 to 20 years: Male 32 to 148 mg/dL, Female 37 to 124 mg/dL.</li></ul>

Total Protein And Fractions

Liver function studies	
Total protein	Determines if the liver is producing protein in normal amounts and evaluates malnutrition: ▯ 0 to 5 days: 3.8 to 6.2 g/dL. ▯ 1-3 years: 5.9 to 7.0 g/dL. ▯ 4-6 years: 5.9 to 7.8 g/dL. ▯ 7 to 9 years: 6.2 to 8.2 g/dL. ▯ 10 to 19 years: 6.3 to 8.6 g/dL. Protein fractions include: **Albumin:**<ul><li>5 days to 14 years: 3.8-5.4 g/dL</li><li>15 to 18 years: 3.2-4.5 g/dL</li></ul>**α1 Globulin:** 0.2 to 0.4 g/dL (Increase in inflammatory diseases). **α2 Globulin:** *0.4 to 0.8 g/dL* (Increase in diabetes, pancreatitis, and hemolysis. Decrease in nephrotic syndrome, chronic inflammatory disorders, and recovery stage of 3ʳᵈ degree burns). **β Globulin:** *0.5 to 1.0 g/dL* (Increase in hyperlipopro-teinemias. Decrease in IgA deficiency and hypo-β-lipoproteinemia). ***Y Globulin:*** 0.6 to 12 g/dL (Increase in liver diseases and chronic infections. Decrease in immune deficiency or immunosuppres-sion)). **Serum protein electrophoresis** is done to determine the ratio of proteins. **Albumin/globulin (A/G) ratio:** 1.5:1 to 2.5:1. (Albumin should be greater than globulin.)

Types of Protein Malnutrition

Protein malnutrition (kwashiorkor or hypoalbuminemia), inadequate protein but adequate fats and carbohydrates, can result from chronic diarrhea, renal disease, infection, hemorrhage, burns, traumatic injuries or other illnesses. Onset is usually rapid with loss of visceral protein while skeletal muscle mass is retained, so it may be difficult to detect on a physical exam.

Symptoms include:
- Hypoalbuminemia and anemia
- Edema
- Delayed healing of wound, immuno-incompetence.

Protein-calorie malnutrition (marasmus), inadequate protein and calories, is usually more obvious. Visceral protein is usually intact as is immune function because weight loss is gradual. However, children are often very thin or emaciated from loss of skeletal muscle mass.

Symptoms include:
- Decreased basal metabolism, hypothermia
- Lack of subcutaneous fat, decreased tissue turgor
- Bradycardia

Mixed protein-calorie malnutrition (combination) is common in hospitalized patients and has an acute onset with low visceral protein as well as rapid loss of weight, skeletal muscle mass, and fat.

Nutritional Lab Monitoring

Albumin
Albumin is a protein that is produced by the liver and is a necessary component for cells and tissues. Levels decrease with renal disease, malnutrition, and severe burns. Albumin levels are the most common screening to determine protein levels. Albumin has a half-life of 18-20 days, so it is sensitive to long-term protein deficiencies more than short-term.

Normal values:
- 5 days to 14 years: 3.8-5.4 g/dL
- 15 to 18 years: 3.2-4.5 g/dL

Levels below 3.2 correlate with increased morbidity and death. Dehydration (poor intake, diarrhea, or vomiting) elevates levels, so adequate hydration is important to ensure meaningful results:
- Mild deficiency: 3-3.5 g/dL
- Moderate deficiency: 2.5-3.0 g/dL
- Severe deficiency: <2.5 g/dL.

Prealbumin
Prealbumin (transthyretin) is most commonly monitored for acute changes in nutritional status because it has a half-life of only 2-3 days. Prealbumin is a protein produced in the

liver, so it is often decreased with liver disease. Amiodarone and diethylstilbesterol can decrease levels. . Levels may rise with Hodgkin's disease or the use of steroids, anticonvulsants, or NSAIDS. Prealbumin is necessary for transportation of both thyroxine and vitamin A throughout the body, so if levels fall, both thyroxine and vitamin A utilization are also affected.

Normal values.
- 0-1 month: 7-39 mg/dL.
- 1-6 months: 8.3-34 mg/dL.
- 6 months to 4 years: 2-36 mg/dL.
- 5-6 years: 12-30 mg/dL.
- 6 years to adult: 12 to 42 mg/dl

Prealbumin is a good measurement because it quickly decreases when nutrition is inadequate and rises quickly in response to increased protein intake. Protein intake must be adequate to maintain levels of prealbumin.

Deficiencies (5 years and older):
- Mild deficiency: 10-15mg/dL
- Moderate deficiency: 5-9 mg/dL.
- Severe deficiency: <5 mg/dL.

Death rates increase with any decrease in prealbumin levels.

Transferrin
Transferrin, which transports about one-third of the body's iron, is a protein produced by the liver. It transports iron from the intestines to the bone marrow where it is used to produce hemoglobin. The half-life of transferrin is about 8-10 days. It is sometimes used as a measure of nutritional status; however, transferrin levels are sensitive to many different things. Levels rapidly decrease with protein malnutrition. Liver disease and anemia can also depress levels, but a decrease in iron, commonly found with inadequate protein, stimulates the liver to produce more transferrin, which increases levels but also decreases production of albumin and prealbumin. Levels may also increase with pregnancy, use of oral contraceptives, and polycythemia. Thus, transferrin levels alone are not always reliable measurements of nutritional status:

Normal values:
- Newborn: 130-275
- Adult: 200-400 mg/dL.
- Mild deficiency: 150-200 mg/dL.
- Moderate deficiency: 100-150 mg/dL.
- Severe deficiency: <100 mg/dL.

Histamine Receptor Antagonists

Histamine (H) receptor antagonists (actually reverse agonists) are used to treat conditions in which excessive stomach acid causes heartburn and GERD. They block histamine 2 (H_2) (parietal) cell receptors in the stomach, thereby decreasing acid production. These drugs are used less commonly now than proton-pump inhibitors.

Common H_2 antagonists include:

- Cimetidine (Tagamet®): The first H_2 antagonist, it is used less frequently than others because of inhibition of enzymes that results in drug interactions, especially with contraceptive agents and estrogen.
- Ranitidine (Zantac®): This was developed to decrease drug interactions and improve patient tolerance. Its activity is about 10 times that of cimetidine. It may be used in combination with other drugs to treat ulcers.
- Famotidine (Pepcid®): This may be combined with an antacid to increase the speed of effects as it has a slow onset. It may be used pre-surgically to reduce post-operative nausea.
- Nizatidine (Axid®): The last H_2 antagonist developed, it is about equal in potency and action to ranitidine.

Serotonin Antagonists

Serotonin antagonists block $5\text{-}HT_2$ receptors of serotonin in the central and peripheral nervous systems and gastrointestinal system. An open channel can result in agitation, nausea, and vomiting, but antagonists close the channel and reduce these symptoms. Serotonin antagonists are frequently used to treat to prevent/treat nausea associated with chemotherapy and anesthesia.

Medications include:

- Metoclopramide (Reglan®) is used to reduce nausea and vomiting from a wide range of causes. It is also a prokinetic drug that increases gastrointestinal contractions and promotes faster gastric emptying, so it is used for heartburn, GERD, and diabetic gastroparesis.
- Ondansetron (Zofran®) reduces vagal stimulation of medulla oblongata (vomiting center) and is used for nausea related to chemotherapy.
- Tropisetron (Navoban®) is used to reduce nausea related to chemotherapy.
- Granisetron (Kytril®) is used to reduce nausea related to chemotherapy, surgery, and radiation.

Serotonin antagonists have fewer side effects than other antiemetics, but may cause muscle cramping, agitation, diarrhea/constipation, dizziness, and headache.

Antacids

Antacids are medications used to reduce stomach acids by raising the pH and neutralizing the acids present. They are commonly used to treat heartburn or indigestion. Adverse reactions are relatively rare unless taken to excess or with renal impairment.

Drugs include:

- Aluminum hydroxide (Amphojel®) may cause constipation and with renal impairment, hypophosphatemia and osteomalacia.
- Magnesium hydroxide (Milk of Magnesia®) (also a laxative) may cause diarrhea and with renal impairment can cause hypermagnesemia.
- Aluminum hydroxide with magnesium hydroxide (Maalox®, Mylanta®).

- Calcium carbonate (TUMS®, Rolaids®, Titralac®) may cause gastric distention. Excess calcium intake may cause toxic reactions, including kidney stones and renal failure; so excess intake should be avoided.
- Alka-Seltzer® combines sodium bicarbonate with aspirin and citric acid so this compound may cause gastric irritation, nausea and vomiting, and tarry stools.
- Bismuth subsalicylate (Pepto-Bismol®). Pepto-Bismol® may react with sulfur in the body to create a black tongue and black stools, but this is temporary. Pepto-Bismol® has been associated with Reye's syndrome in children with influenza or chickenpox.

Proton Pump Inhibitors

Proton pump inhibitors (PPIs) are now used more frequently than histamine receptor antagonists. PPIs interfere with an acid-producing enzyme in the stomach wall, reducing stomach acid. PPIs are used to treat GERD, stomach ulcers, and *H. pylori* (with antibiotics). PPIs are similar in action and include:
- Esomeprazole (Nexium®)
- Lansoprazole (Prevacid®)
- Omeprazole (Prilosec®)
- Pantoprazole (Protonix®)
- Rabeprazole (Aciphex®)
- Omeprazole/sodium bicarbonate (Zegerid®) (Long-acting form of omeprazole.

Common side effects include gastrointestinal upset (nausea, diarrhea, constipation), headache, and rash. In rare instances, PPIs may cause severe muscle pain; however, they are usually well-tolerated with few adverse effects. PPIs may interfere with the absorption of some drugs, such as those that are affected by stomach acid. Absorption of ketoconazole is impaired, and absorption of digoxin is increased, sometimes leading to toxicity. Omeprazole impacts the hepatic breakdown of drugs more than other PPIs and may cause increased levels of diazepam, phenytoin, and warfarin.

Renal

Acute renal failure

Acute renal failure is abrupt and almost complete failure of kidney function with decreased glomerular filtration rate (GFR), occurring over a period of hours/days. It most commonly occurs in hospitalized patients but may occur in others as well. The BUN increases and nitrogenous wastes are retained (azotemia). There are 3 primary categories, related to cause:

- Prerenal disorders, such as myocardial infraction, heart failure, sepsis, anaphylaxis, and hemorrhage result in hypoperfusion of the kidney and ↓ GFR.
- Intrarenal disorders include burns, trauma, infection, transfusion reactions, and nephrotoxic agents that cause damage to glomeruli or kidney tubules, such as acute tubular necrosis. Burns and crush trauma injuries release myoglobin and hemoglobin from tissues, causing renal toxicity and/or ischemia. With transfusion reactions, hemolysis occurs, and the broken down hemoglobin concentrates and precipitates in tubules. Medications, such as NSAIDs and ACE inhibitors may interfere with kidney function and cause hypoperfusion and ischemia.
- Post renal disorders involve distal obstruction that increases pressure in tubules and ↓ GFR.

Acute Tubular Necrosis

Acute tubular necrosis (ATN) occurs when a hypoxic condition causes renal ischemia that damages tubular cells of the glomeruli so they are unable to adequately filter the urine, leading to acute renal failure. Causes include hypotension, hyperbilirubinemia, sepsis, surgery (especially cardiac or vascular), and birth complications. ATN may result from nephrotoxic injury related to obstruction or drugs, such as chemotherapy, acyclovir, and antibiotics, such as sulfonamides and streptomycin. Symptoms may be non-specific initially and can include life-threatening complications.

Symptoms	Treatment
Lethargy. Nausea and vomiting. Hypovolemia with low cardiac output and generalized vasodilation. Fluid and electrolyte imbalance leading to hypertension, CNS abnormalities, metabolic acidosis, arrhythmias, edema, and congestive heart failure. Uremia leading to destruction of platelets and bleeding, neurological deficits, and disseminated intravascular coagulopathy (DIC). Infections can include pericarditis and sepsis.	Identifying and treating underlying cause. Supportive care. Loop diuretics (in some cases), such as Lasix®. Antibiotics for infection. Discontinuation of nephrotoxic agents. Dopamine (low dose) to increase renal circulation, Kidney dialysis. Restricting potassium and phosphate.

Loop Diuretics

Diuretics increase renal perfusion and filtration, thereby reducing preload and decreasing peripheral and pulmonary edema, hypertension, CHF, diabetes insipidus, and osteoporosis. There are different types of diuretics: loop, thiazide, and potassium sparing.

Loop diuretics inhibit the reabsorption of sodium and chloride (primarily) in the ascending loop of Henle. They also cause increased secretion of other electrolytes, such as calcium, magnesium, and potassium, and this can result in imbalances that cause dysrhythmias. Other side effects include frequent urination, postural hypotension, and increased blood sugar and uric acid levels. They are short-acting so are less effective than other diuretics for control of hypertension:

- Bumetanide (Bumex®) is given intravenously after surgery to reduce preload or orally to treat heart failure.
- Ethacrynic acid (Edecrin®) is given intravenously after surgery to reduce preload.
- Furosemide (Lasix®) is used for the control of congestive heart failure as well as renal insufficiency. It is used after surgery to decrease preload and to reduce the inflammatory response caused by cardiopulmonary bypass (post-perfusion syndrome).

Thiazide Diuretics

Thiazide diuretics inhibit the reabsorption of sodium and chloride primarily in the early distal tubules, forcing more sodium and water to be excreted. Thiazide diuretics increase secretion of potassium and bicarbonate, so they are often given with supplementary potassium or in combination with potassium-sparing diuretics. Thiazide diuretics are the first line of drugs for treatment of hypertension. They have a long duration of action (12-72 hours, depending on the drug) so they are able to maintain control of hypertension better than short-acting drugs. They may be given daily or 3-5 days per week. There are numerous thiazide diuretics, including:

- Chlorothiazide (Diuril®)
- Bendroflumethiazide (Naturetin®)
- Chlorthalidone (Hygroton)
- Trichlormethiazide (Naqua®)

Side effects include dizziness, lightheadedness, postural hypotension, headache, blurred vision, and itching, especially during initial treatment. Thiazide diuretics cause sensitivity to sun exposure, so people should be counseled to use sunscreen.

Potassium-Sparing Diuretics

Potassium-sparing diuretics inhibit the reabsorption of sodium in the late distal tubule and collecting duct. They are weaker than thiazide or loop diuretics, but do not cause a reduction in potassium level; however, if used alone, they may cause an increase in potassium, which can cause weakness, irregular pulse, and cardiac arrest. Because potassium-sparing diuretics are less effective alone, they are often given in a combined form with a thiazide diuretic (usually chlorothiazide), which mitigates the potassium imbalance. Typical side effects include dehydration, blurred vision, nausea insomnia, and nasal congestion, especially in the first few days of treatment:

- Spironolactone (Aldactone®) is a synthetic steroid diuretic that increases the secretion of both water and sodium and is used to treat congestive heart failure. It may be given orally or intravenously.
- Eplerenone is similar to spironolactone but has fewer side effects so it may be used with patients who can't tolerate the other drug.

End-Stage Renal Disease

End-stage (chronic) renal disease (ESRD) occurs with chronic renal failure when the kidneys are unable to filter and excrete wastes, concentrate urine, and maintain electrolyte balance because of hypoxic conditions, kidney disease, or obstruction in the urinary tract. It results first in azotemia (increase in nitrogenous waste in the blood) and then in uremia (nitrogenous wastes cause toxic symptoms.) When >50% of the functional renal capacity is destroyed, the kidneys can no longer carry out necessary functions and progressive deterioration begins over months or years. Symptoms are often non-specific in the beginning with loss of appetite and energy.

Symptoms and complications	Treatment
Weight loss. Headaches, muscle cramping, general malaise. Increased bruising and dry or itching skin. Increased BUN and creatinine. Sodium and fluid retention with edema. Hyperkalemia. Metabolic acidosis. Calcium and phosphorus depletion, resulting in altered bone metabolism, pain, and retarded growth. Anemia with decreased production on RBCs. Increased risk of infection. Uremic syndrome.	Supportive/symptomatic therapy. Dialysis and transplantation. Diet control: Low protein, salt, potassium, and phosphorus. Fluid limitations. Calcium and vitamin supplementation. Phosphate binders.

Uremic Syndrome
Uremic syndrome is a number of disorders that can occur with end-stage renal disease and renal failure, usually after multiple metabolic failures and decrease in creatinine clearance to <10mL/min. There is compromise of all normal functions of the kidney: fluid balance, electrolyte balance, acid-base homeostasis, hormone production, and elimination of wastes. Metabolic abnormalities related to uremia include:
- Decreased RBC production: The kidney is unable to produce adequate erythropoietin in the peritubular cells, resulting in anemia, which is usually normocytic and normochromic. Parathyroid hormone levels may increase, causing calcification of the bone marrow, causing hypoproliferative anemia as RBC production is suppressed.
- Platelet abnormalities: Decreased platelet count, increased turnover, and reduced adhesion lead to bleeding disorders.
- Metabolic acidosis: The tubular cells are unable to regulate acid-base metabolism, and phosphate, sulfuric, hippuric, and lactic acids increase, leading to congestive heart failure and weakness.
- Hyperkalemia: The nephrons cannot excrete adequate amounts of potassium. Some drugs, such as diuretics that spare potassium may aggravate the condition.

<u>Renal Bone Disease, Multiple Endocrine Disorders, Cardiovascular Disorders, Anorexia And Malnutrition</u>

Metabolic abnormalities associated with end-stage renal disease and uremic syndrome include:

- Renal bone disease: Decreased calcium, increased phosphate and parathyroid hormone, decreased utilization of vitamin D lead to demineralization. In some cases, calcium and phosphate are deposited in other tissues (metastatic calcification).

- Multiple endocrine disorders: Thyroid hormone production is decreased and reproductive hormones abnormalities may result in infertility/impotence. Males have decreased testosterone but increased estrogen and LH. Females experience irregular cycles, lack of ovulation and menses. Insulin production may increase but with decreased clearance, resulting in episodes of hypoglycemia or decreased hyperglycemia in those who are diabetic.
- Cardiovascular disorders: Left ventricular hypertrophy is most common, but fluid retention may cause congestive heart failure and electrolyte imbalances, dysrhythmias. Pericarditis, exacerbation of valvular disorders, and pericardial effusions may occur.
- Anorexia and malnutrition: Nausea and poor appetite contribute to hypoalbuminemia, sometimes exacerbated by restrictive diets.

Renal Dialysis

<u>Peritoneal Dialysis</u>

Renal dialysis is used primarily for those who have progressed from renal insufficiency to uremia with end stage renal disease (ESRD). It may also be temporarily for acute conditions. Children can be maintained on dialysis, but there are many complications associated with dialysis so many children are considered for renal transplantation. There are a number of different approaches to dialysis:

- Peritoneal dialysis: An indwelling catheter is inserted surgically into the peritoneal cavity with a subcutaneous tunnel and a Dacron cuff to prevent infection. Sterile dialysate solution is slowly instilled through gravity, remains for a prescribed length of time, and is then drained and discarded.
- Continuous ambulatory peritoneal dialysis: A series of exchange cycles are repeated 24 hours a day.
- Continuous cyclic peritoneal dialysis: A prolonged period of retaining fluid occurs during the day with drainage at night.

Peritoneal dialysis may be used for those who want to be more independent, don't live near a dialysis center, or want fewer dietary restrictions.

<u>Hemodialysis</u>

Hemodialysis, the most common type of dialysis, is used for both short-term dialysis and long-term for those with ESRD. Treatments are usually done 3 times weekly for 3-4 hours or short daily dialysis with treatment either during the night or in short daily periods. Hemodialysis is often done for those who can't manage peritoneal dialysis or who live near a dialysis center, but it does interfere with work or school attendance and requires strict dietary and fluid restrictions between treatments. Short daily dialysis allows more independence, and increased costs may be offset by lower morbidity. A vascular access device, such as a catheter, fistula, or graft must be established for hemodialysis, and heparin is used to prevent clotting. With hemodialysis, blood is circulated outside of the body through a dialyzer (a synthetic semipermeable membrane), which filters the blood. There are many different types of dialyzers. High flux dialyzers use a highly permeable membrane that shortens the duration of treatment and decreases the need for heparin.

Continuous Renal Replacement Therapy

Continuous renal replacement therapy (CCRT) circulates the blood by hydrostatic pressure through a semipermeable membrane. It is used in critical care and can be instituted quickly:

- Continuous arteriovenous hemofiltration (CAVH) circulates blood from an artery (usually the femoral) to a hemofilter using only arterial pressure and not a blood pump. The filtered blood is then returned to the patients venous system, often with added fluids to offset those lost. Only the fluid in filtered.
- Continuous arteriovenous hemodialysis (CAVHD) is similar to CAVH except that dialysate circulates on one side of the semipermeable membrane to increase clearance of urea.
- Continuous venovenous hemofiltration (CVVH) pumps blood through a double-lumen venous catheter to a hemofilter, which returns the blood to the patient in the same catheter. It provides continuous slow removal of fluid, is better tolerated with unstable patients, and doesn't require arterial access.

Continuous venovenous hemodialysis is similar to CVVH but uses a dialysate to increase clearance of uremic toxins.

Complications Associated With Dialysis

There are many complications associated with dialysis, especially when used for long-term treatment:

- Hemodialysis: Long-term use promotes atherosclerosis and cardiovascular disease. Anemia and fatigue are common as are infections related to access devices or contamination of equipment. Some experience hypotension and muscle cramping during treatment. Dysrhythmias may occur. Some may exhibit dialysis disequilibrium from cerebral fluid shifts, causing headaches, nausea and vomiting, and alterations of consciousness.
- Peritoneal dialysis: Most complications are minor, but it can lead to peritonitis, which requires removal of the catheter if antibiotic therapy is not successful in clearing the infection within 4 days. There may be leakage of the dialysate around the catheter. Bleeding may occur, especially in females who are menstruating as blood is pulled from the uterus through the fallopian tubes. Abdominal hernias may occur with long use. Some may have anorexia from feeling of fullness or sweet taste in mouth from absorption of glucose.

Fluid Balance/Fluid Deficit

Body fluid is primarily intracellular fluid (ICF) or extracellular space (ECF). By 3 years of age, the fluid balance has stabilized and remains throughout adulthood:

- ECF: 20-30% (intrastitial fluid, plasma, transcellular fluid).

- ICF: 40-50% (fluid within the cells)

The fluid compartments are separated by semipermeable membranes that allow fluid and solutes (electrolytes and other substances) to move by osmosis. Fluid also moves through diffusion, filtration, and active transport. In fluid volume deficit, fluid is out of balance and ECF is depleted; an overload occurs with increased concentration of sodium and retention of fluid.

Signs of fluid deficit include:
- Thirsty, restless to lethargic.
- Increasing pulse rate, tachycardia.
- Fontanels depressed (infants).
- Decreased urinary output.
- Normal BP progressing hypotension.
- Dry mucous membranes
- 3-10% decrease in body weight.

Electrolyte Imbalances

Sodium
Sodium (Na) regulates fluid volume, osmolality, acid-base balance, and activity in the muscles, nerves and myocardium. It is the primary cation (positive ion) in ECF, necessary to maintain ECF levels that are needed for tissue perfusion:
- Normal value: Infant 133 to 144 mEq/L, Child 135-145 mEq/L
- Hyponatremia: <133 to 135 mEq/L.
- Hypernatremia: >145 mEq/L.

Hypo-natremia	May result from inadequate sodium intake or excess loss, through diarrhea, vomiting, NG suctioning. It can occur as the result of illness, such as severe burns, fever, SIADH, and ketoacidosis. Symptoms vary: ▢ Irritability to lethargy to lethargy and alterations in consciousness. ▢ Cerebral edema with seizures and coma. ▢ Dyspnea to respiratory failure. *Treatment:* Identify and treat underlying cause and provide Na replacement.
Hyper-natremia	May result from renal disease, diabetes insipidus, and fluid depletion. *Symptoms* include irritability to lethargy to confusion to coma, seizures, flushing, muscle weakness and spasms, and thirst. *Treatment* includes identifying and treating underlying cause, monitoring Na levels carefully, and IV fluid replacement.

Potassium Depletion
Potassium (K) is the primary electrolyte in ICF with about 98% inside cells and only 2% in ECF, although this small amount is important for neuromuscular activity. K influences activity of the skeletal and cardiac muscles. K level is dependent upon adequate renal functioning because 80% is excreted through the kidneys and 20% through the bowels and sweat:

- Normal values: Infant 4.1 to 5.3 mEq/L, Child 3.4 to 4.7 mEq/L
- Hypokalemia: <3.4 mEq/L (age dependent). Critical value: <2.5 mEq/L

Hypo-kalemia	Caused by loss of K through diarrhea, vomiting, gastric suction, and diuresis, alkalosis, decreased K intake with starvation, and nephritis. *Symptoms* include: • Lethargy and weakness. • Nausea and vomiting. • Paresthesias. • Dysrhythmias with EKG abnormalities: PVCs, flattened T waves. • Muscle cramps with hyporeflexia. • Hypotension. • Tetany. *Treatment:* Identify and treat underlying cause and replace K.

Potassium Excess

Hyper-kalemia >5.5 mEq/L. Critical value: >6.5 mEq/L	Caused by renal disease, adrenal insufficiency, metabolic acidosis, severe dehydration, burns, hemolysis, and trauma. It rarely occurs without renal disease but may be induced by treatment (such as NSAIDs and potassium-sparing diuretics). Untreated renal failure results in reduced excretion. Those with Addison's disease and deficient adrenal hormones suffer sodium loss that results in potassium retention. The primary symptoms relates to the effect on the cardiac muscle: ⬚ Ventricular arrhythmias with increasing changes in EKC leading to cardiac and respiratory arrest. ⬚ Weakness with ascending paralysis and hyperreflexia. ⬚ Diarrhea. ⬚Increasing confusion. *Treatment* includes identifying underlying cause and discontinuing sources of increased K: ⬚ Calcium gluconate to decrease cardiac effects. ⬚ Sodium bicarbonate shifts K into the cells temporarily. ⬚ Insulin and hypertonic dextrose shift K into the cells temporarily. ⬚ Cation exchange resin (Kayexalate®) to decrease K. ⬚ Peritoneal dialysis or hemodialysis

Calcium

More than 99% of calcium (Ca) is in the skeletal system with 1% in serum, but it is important for transmitting nerve impulses and regulating muscle contraction and relaxation, including the myocardium. Calcium activates enzymes that stimulate chemical reactions and has a role in coagulation of blood:

- Normal values: 11 days to 2 years: 9 to 11 mg/dL. 3 to 12 years: 8.8 to 10.8 mg/dL. 13 to 18 years: 8.4 to 10.2 mg/dL.
- Hypocalcemia: <8.4 mg/dL. Critical value: <7 mg/dL.
- Hypercalcemia: Age-dependent. Critical value: >12 mg/dL.

Hypo-calcemia	May be caused by hypoparathyroidism and occurs after thyroid and parathyroid surgery, pancreatitis, renal failure, inadequate vitamin D, alkalosis, magnesium deficiency and low serum albumin. Symptoms include: Tetany, tingling, seizures, altered mental status. Ventricular tachycardia. Treatment: Calcium replacement and vitamin D.
Hyper-calcemia	May be caused by acidosis, kidney disease, hyperparathyroidism, prolonged immobilization, and malignancies. Crisis carries a 50% mortality rate. Symptoms include: Increasing muscle weakness with hypotonicity. Anorexia, nausea and vomiting. Constipation. Bradycardia and cardiac arrest. Treatment: Identify and treat underlying cause, loop diuretics, and IV fluids.

Phosphorus

Phosphorus, or phosphate, (PO_4) is necessary for neuromuscular and red blood cell function, the maintenance of acid-base balance, and provides structure for teeth and bones. About 85% is in the bones, 14% in soft tissue, and <1% in ECF. Normal values:

1-3 years: 3.9-6.5 mg/dL.	12 to 13 years: 3.3 to 5.4 mg/dL.
4-6 years: 4.0-5.4 mg/dL.	14 to 15 years: 2.9 to 5.4 mg/dL.
7-11 years: 3.7-5.6 mg/dL.	16 to 19 years: 2.8 to 4.6 mg/dL.
Hypophos-phatemia Critical value: <1 mg/dL.	Occurs with severe protein-calorie malnutrition, excess antacids with magnesium, calcium or albumin, hyperventilation, severe burns, and diabetic ketoacidosis. *Symptoms* include: Irritability, tremors, seizures to coma. Hemolytic anemia. Decreased myocardial function. Respiratory failure. *Treatment:* Identify and treat underlying cause and replace phosphorus.
Hyper-phos-phatemia	Occurs with renal failure, hypoparathyroidism, excessive intake, and neoplastic disease, diabetic ketoacidosis, muscle necrosis, and chemotherapy. *Symptoms* include: Tachycardia. Muscle cramping, hyperreflexia, and tetany. Nausea and diarrhea. *Treatment:* Identify and treat underlying cause, correct hypocalcemia, and provide antacids and dialysis.

Magnesium

Magnesium (Mg) is the second most common intracellular electrolyte (after potassium) and activates many intracellular enzyme systems. Mg is important for carbohydrate and protein metabolism, neuromuscular function, and cardiovascular function, producing vasodilation and directly affecting the peripheral arterial system.

Normal values (Child): 1.7 to 2.1 mEq/L.

Hypomagnesemia: <1.7 mEq/L. Critical value: <1.2 mg/dL.

Hypermagnesemia: >2.1 mEq/L. Critical value: >4.9 mg/dL.

Hypo-magnes-emia	Occurs with chronic diarrhea, chronic renal disease, chronic pancreatitis, excess diuretic or laxative use, hyperthyroidism, hypoparathyroidism, severe burns, and diaphoresis. *Symptoms* include: Neuro-muscular excitability/ tetany. Confusion, headaches & dizzy-ness, seizure and coma. Tachycardia with ventricular arrhythmias. Respiratory depression. *Treatment:* Identify and treat underlying cause, provide magnesium replacement.
Hyper-mag-nesemia	Occurs with renal failure or inadequate renal function, diabetic ketoacidosis, hypothyroidism, and Addison's disease. *Symptoms* include muscle weakness, seizures, and dysphagia with decreased gag reflex, tachycardia with hypotension. *Treatment:* Identify and treat underlying cause, IV hydration with calcium, and dialysis.

Metabolic and Respiratory Acidosis

Pathophysiology –
Metabolic - Increase in fixed acid and inability to excrete acid or loss of base, with compensatory increase of CO_2 excretion by lungs.

Respiratory - Hypoventilation and CO_2 retention, with renal compensatory retention of bicarbonate (HCO_3) and increased excretion of hydrogen.

Laboratory –
Metabolic - Decreased serum pH and PCO_2 normal if uncompensated and decreased if compensated. Decreased HCO_3.
Urine pH <6 if compensated.

Respiratory - Increased serum pH and increased PCO_2. Increased HCO_3 if compensated and normal if uncompensated. Urine pH >6 if compensated.

Causes –
Metabolic - DKA, lactic acidosis, diarrhea, starvation, renal failure, shock, renal tubular acidosis, starvation

Respiratory - COPD, overdose of sedative or barbiturate, obesity, severe pneumonia/atelectasis, muscle weakness (Guillain-Barré), mechanical hypoventilation.

Symptoms –
Metabolic -Neuro/muscular: drowsiness, confusion headache, coma. Cardiac: Decreased BP, arrhythmias, flushed skin.
GI: nausea, vomiting, abdominal pain, diarrhea.
Respiratory: Deep inspired tachypnea.

Respiratory - Neuro/muscular: drowsiness, dizziness, headache, coma, disorientation, seizures. Cardiac: Flushed skin, VF, decreased BP
GI: absent. Respiratory: Hypoventilation with hypoxia.

Metabolic and Respiratory Alkalosis

Pathophysiology –
Metabolic - Decreased strong acid or increased base, with compensatory CO_2 retention by lungs.

Respiratory - Hyperventilation and increased excretion of CO_2, with compensatory HCO_3 excretion by kidneys.

Laboratory –
Metabolic -Increased serum pH. PCO_2 normal if uncompensated and increased if compensated. Increased HCO_3 Urine pH >6 if compensated.

Respiratory - Increased serum pH. Decreased PCO_2. HCO_3 normal if uncompen-sated and decreased if compensated. Urine pH >6 if compensated.
Causes -
Metabolic - Excessive vomiting, gastric suctioning, diuretics, potassium deficit, excessive mineralocorticoids and $NaHCO_3$ intake.

Respiratory - Hyperventilation associated with hypoxia, pulmonary embolus, exercise, anxiety, pain, and fever.
Encephalopathy, septicemia, brain injury, salicylate overdose, mechanical hyperventilation.

Symptoms –
Metabolic - Neuro/muscular: dizziness, confusion, nervousness, anxiety, tremors, muscle cramping, tetany, tingling, seizures. Cardiac: Tachycardia and arrhythmias. GI: Nausea, vomiting, anorexia. Respiratory: Compensatory hypoventilation.

Respiratory Neuro/muscular: Light-headed, confused, and lethargic.
Cardiac: Tachycardia and arrhythmias. GI: Epigastric pain, nausea and vomiting.
Respiratory: Hyperventilation.

Hydronephrosis

Hydronephrosis is a symptom of a disease involving swelling of the kidney pelvises and calyces because of an obstruction that causes urine to be retained in the kidney. In chronic conditions, symptoms may be delayed until severe kidney damage has occurred. Over time, the kidney begins to atrophy. The primary condition conditions that predispose to hydronephrosis include:

- Vesicoureteral reflux.
- Obstruction at the ureteropelvic junction.
- Renal edema (non-obstructive).

Any condition that impairs drainage of the ureters can cause backup of the urine.

Symptoms	Treatment
• Symptoms vary widely depending upon cause and whether the condition is acute or chronic. • Acute episodes are usually characterized by flank pain, abnormal creatinine and electrolyte levels, and increased pH. • The enlarged kidney may be palpable as a soft mass	• Treatment requires identifying the cause of obstruction and correcting it to ensure adequate drainage. • A nephrostomy tube, ureteral stent or pyeloplasty may be done surgically in some cases. • A urinary catheter may be inserted if there is outflow obstruction from the bladder.

Renal Trauma

Most renal trauma in children is the result of blunt trauma associated with motor vehicle accidents, falls, sports injuries, and child abuse although gunshot wounds and stabbings also occur with increasing frequency. Various staging systems are used, but overall injuries are graded by severity:

A. Contusion of cortex with fracture (tear) of small confined area.
B. Major fracture with peri-renal hematoma and/or extravasation of urine.
C. Multiple fractures with extensive bleeding.
D. Severe vascular disruption decreasing perfusion of kidney.

Symptoms	Treatment

Kidney injuries are often accompanied by other trauma (75%) so symptoms may be complex:
• Pain in abdominal or flank area.
• Hematuria.
• Abrasions or contusions in flank or abdominal area.
• Shock.
• Delayed symptoms include hypertension, hydronephrosis.
	• Treatment is usually non-operative if the child is hemodynamically stable, based on evaluation by CT, especially for blunt trauma.
	  o Bed rest.
	  o Monitoring of blood counts and vital signs.
	• Gunshot wounds usually require surgical exploration.

Urinalysis

Urinalysis	
Color	Pale yellow/ amber and darkens when urine is concentrated or other substances (such as blood or bile) or present.
Appearance	Clear but may be slightly cloudy.
Odor	Slight. Bacteria may give urine a foul smell, depending upon the organism. Some foods, such as asparagus, change odor.
Specific gravity	1.015 to 1.025. May increase if protein levels increase or if there is fever, vomiting, or dehydration.
pH	Usually ranges between 4.5 to 8 with average of 5 to 6.

Sediment	Red cell casts from acute infections, broad casts from kidney disorders, and white cell casts from pyelonephritis. Leukocytes > 10 per ml^3 are present with urinary tract infections.
Glucose, ketones, protein, blood, bilirubin, and nitrate	Negative. Urine glucose may increase with infection (with normal blood glucose). Frank blood may be caused by some parasites and diseases but also by drugs, smoking, excessive exercise, and menstrual fluids. Increased red blood cells may result from lower urinary tract infections.
Urobilinogen	0.1-1.0 units.

Renal Function Studies

Spgr, Urine And Serum Osmolality, Serum And Urine Uric Acid, And BUN

Renal function studies	
Specific gravity	1.015-1.025. Determines kidney's ability to concentrate urinary solutes.
Osmolality (urine)	250-900 mOsm/kg/24 hours. Shows early defects if kidney's ability to concentrate urine is impaired.
Osmolality (serum)	275-295 mOsm/kg.
Uric acid (serum)	• 0 to 12 years: 2.0 to 5.5 mg/dL. • 13 to adult: Male 4.4 to 7.6, Female 2.3 to 6.6. Levels increase with renal failure.
Uric acid (urine)	• Male: 250 to 800 mg/24 hr. • Female: 250 to 750 mg/24 hr.
Blood urea nitrogen (BUN)	• 0 to 3 years: 5 to 17 mg/dL. • 4 to 13 years: 7 to 17 mg/dL. • 14 to adulthood: 8 to 21 mg/dL. Increase indicates impaired renal function, as urea is end product of protein metabolism.

BUN/Creatinine Ratio, Creatinine Clearance, And Serum And Urine Creatinine

Renal function studies	
BUN/creatine ratio	10:1. Increases with hypovolemia. With intrinsic kidney disease, the ratio is normal, but the BUN and creatinine are increased.
Creatinine clearance, 24-hour (urine)	• Children: 70 to 140 mL/min/1.73 m^2. Evaluates the amount of blood cleared of creatinine in 1 minute. Approximates the glomerular filtration rate.
Creatinine (serum)	• 1 to 5 years: 0.3 to 05 mg/dL. • 6 to 10 years: 0.5 to 0.8 mg/dL. • To adulthood: Male 0.6 to 12 mg/dL, Female 0.5 to 1.1 mg/dL. Increases with impaired renal function, urinary tract obstruction, and nephritis. Level should remain stable with normal functioning.
Creatinine	• 2 to 3 years: 6 to 22 mg/kg/24 hr.

(urine)	• 4 to 18 years: 12 to 30 mg/kg/24 hr.

Intravenous Pyelogram

Intravenous pyelogram (IVP) is done to identify structural defects and tumors and to observe urinary structures. The child is administered an IV contrast medium and may be administered antihistamine or corticosteroid before test to minimize allergic response. Serum creatinine and BUN are done prior to the IVP to ensure that the contrast medium can be excreted. During the procedure, radiographs are taken every minute x 5 and then after 15 minutes (giving the contrast medium time to pass into the bladder). A post-voiding radiograph shows how efficient the bladder is in emptying. Fluid intake should be increased post-procedure to flush contrast.

Radionucleotide Renal Scan

Radionucleotide renal scan with dimercaptosuccinic acid (DMSA) requires IV administration of a radioactive element followed by a series of CT scans taken over 20 minutes to 4 hours. The scan is used to assess function and perfusion of the kidney and can detect lesions, atrophy and scars and differentiate among different causes for hydronephrosis. The child must be well hydrated and may need to be catheterized to measure output of urine.

Radical Nephrectomy

Radical nephrectomy is done for adenocarcinoma of the kidney, which may be associated with paraneoplastic syndromes. Some patients have erythrocytosis, but many are anemic and may require transfusions in preparation for surgery to increase hemoglobin to >10 g/dL. Surgery is done under endotracheal general anesthesia with an anterior subcostal, flank, or thoracoabdominal (preferred for large tumors) incision. The kidney and its adrenal gland with surrounding fat and fascia are removed together. Blood loss may be extensive because the tumors tend to be vascular and large, requiring multiple transfusions. However, controlled hypotension should be limited to brief periods because it may impair renal function. Mannitol is given prior to dissection. Continual direct arterial pressure monitoring and central venous cannulation must be done.

Nephron-sparing surgery (partial nephrectomy), often by laparoscopy, may be done if the renal cell carcinoma is <4 cm diameter. Postoperative analgesia and pulmonary hygiene are essential.

Renal Biopsy

Renal biopsy to remove a small segment of cortical tissue helps to identify the extent of kidney disease with acute renal failure, transplant rejection, glomerulopathies, and persistent hematuria or proteinuria. Preoperative coagulation studies determine risk of bleeding. Biopsy is done percutaneously per needle biopsy (guided by fluoroscopy or ultrasound) or surgically through a small flank incision. A urine specimen must be obtained so it can be compared with a post-procedure specimen.

Post-procedure:

- Maintain patient in prone position immediately after procedure and on bedrest for 6 to 8 hours. Monitor urine for hematuria and compare with preop specimen.
- Monitor VS every 5 to 15 minutes for first hour and then less frequently, noting hypotension, tachycardia.
- Note anorexia, vomiting, abdominal discomfort that suggest bleeding.
- Note pain: Severe colicky pain may indicate clot in the ureter.
- Obtain hemoglobin and hematocrit levels within 8 hours.
- Maintain fluid intake at 3000 mL/day in absence of renal insufficiency.
- Provide blood component therapy and surgical repair if bleeding occurs.

Renal Ultrasound

Renal ultrasound is a non-invasive method of viewing the urinary structures. Ultrasound uses ultrasonic sound waves transmitted by a transducer, which picks up reflected sound waves that a computer converts to electronic images. Ultrasound can show fluid accumulation, the movement of blood through the kidney, masses, malformations (congenital abnormalities), and changes in size of the kidney or other structures, and obstructions, such as renal calculi. Ultrasound is usually done before a renal biopsy, and may be done with a needle biopsy to guide placement of needle. Patient preparation includes drinking two 8-ounce glasses of water one hour before the examination to ensure that the bladder is full. The patient should be reminded not to urinate before the ultrasound. The patient usually remains in supine position throughout the procedure but may be asked to turn to the side. No special precautions are necessary post-procedure.

Ureteropelvic Junction Obstruction

Ureteropelvic junction obstruction (UPI) is congenital obstruction at the point where the ureter connects to the renal pelvis, unilaterally or bilaterally, causing inadequate urinary flow and hydronephrosis. Some neonates improve markedly within first 18 months, but others require early surgical repair.

Diagnosis is based on:

- Fetal ultrasound: In utero diagnosis.
- Renal ultrasound: To show dilation of renal pelvis.
- Intravenous pyelogram (IVP): To identify obstruction.
- Renal isotope scan: To evaluate and measure kidney function.

Symptoms	Treatment
• Urinary tract infections. • Inadequate urine output. • Abdominal or flank pain • Palpable mass from hydronephrosis. • Vomiting.	• **Pyeloplasty**: Open surgical procedure where ureteropelvic junction is excised and ureter reattached to renal pelvis with wide junction, allowing adequate drainage. • **Laparoscopic pyeloplasty:** Through abdominal wall and abdominal cavity with internal excision of ureteropelvic junction. • **Insertion of wire through ureter:** To cut ureteropelvic junction from inside with a ureteral drain left in place for a few weeks.

Multisystem

Traumatic Asphyxia and Strangulation

Asphyxia may relate to a number of different injuries:
- Traumatic asphyxia most commonly involves a crush injury of the thorax, and traumatic injuries to multiple organs may be present. Crush injuries are characterized by petechiae in the area of compression although tight-fitting clothing, such as a girl's bra, may prevent petechiae from forming.
- Manual strangulation may involve crush injuries to the throat, such as hyoid fracture. Often the face appears cyanotic while the rest of the body does not. Petechiae may be present on the face as well. Bruising may be noted about the throat.
- Ligature strangulation is similar to manual although throat markings are different, with an indented area surrounding the neck.

- Hanging produces a V-shaped marking on the throat and does not encircle the neck.
- Choking obstructs the airway. (May require bronchoscopy to remove foreign object).

In all cases, immediate establishment of airway, breathing, and circulation (ABCs) takes precedence. Surgical intervention may be needed for traumatic crush injuries.

Distributive Shock

Distributive shock occurs with adequate blood volume but inadequate intravascular volume because of arterial/venous dilation that results in decreased vascular tone and hypoperfusion of internal organs. Cardiac output may be normal or blood may pool, decreas-ing cardiac output. Distributive shock may result from anaphylactic shock, septic shock, neurogenic shock, and drug ingestions:

Symptoms	Treatment

• Hypotension (age-dependent), tachypnea, tachycardia (age-dependent). BP may be lower if patient receiving β-blockers.
• Skin initially warm, later hypo-perfused.
• Hyper- or hypothermia (>38ºC or <36ºC).
• Hypoxemia.
• Alterations in mentation.
• Decreased Urinary output.
• Symptoms related to underlying cause.
	• Treating underlying cause and stabilizing hemodynamics:
	  o Septic shock or anaphylactic therapy and monitoring as indicated.
	  o Oxygen with endotracheal intubation if necessary.
	• Rapid fluid administration at 20 mL/kg NS (sometimes up to 40 to 60 mL/kg) over 20 to 30 minutes or isotonic crystalloid every 5-10 minutes as needed.
	• Albumin 4 to 5 mL/kg over 30 minutes to maintain cardiac output.
	• Inotropic agents (dopamine, dobutamine, norepinephrine) if necessary,

Anaphylaxis Syndrome

Anaphylaxis syndrome may present with a few symptoms or a wide range that encompasses cardiopulmonary, dermatological, and gastrointestinal responses. Symptoms may recur after the initial treatment (biphasic anaphylaxis) in about 6% of children, so careful monitoring is essential:

Symptoms	Treatment
Sudden onset of weakness, dizziness, confusion. Severe generalized edema and angioedema. Lips and tongue may swell. Urticaria Increased permeability of vascular system and loss of vascular tone. Severe hypotension leading to shock. Laryngospasm/bronchospasm with obstruction of airway causing dyspnea and wheezing. Nausea, vomiting, and diarrhea. Seizures, coma and death.	Establish patent airway and intubate if necessary for ventilation. Provide oxygen at 100% high flow. Monitor VS. Administer epinephrine (Epi-pen® or 1:1000 solution 0.1mg/kg to maximum 0.3 mg). Albuterol 2.5 mg (or 0.5%) per nebulizer for bronchospasm Intravenous fluids to provide bolus of fluids for hypotension. Diphenhydramine 1.0 mg/kg (to maximum of 50 mg) if shock persists. Methylprednisolone 2.0 mg/kg if no response to other drugs.

Hemolytic Uremic Syndrome

Hemolytic uremic syndrome is a life-threatening disorder usually follows an *E. coli* infection.

Symptoms	Treatment
• Weakness, lethargy. • Nausea and increased diarrhea. • Fever. • Hematuria and decreased urinary output. • Petechiae and ecchymosis. • Blood in the stool • Jaundice. • Alterations in consciousness. • Seizures (rare). • Bleeding from the nose or mouth occurs as platelets decrease and clotting time increases. • Hypertension. • Edema. • Paralysis (cerebral blood clot).	• Antibiotics are contraindicated unless sepsis is present because they may increase release of toxins associated with *E. coli*. • Intravenous fluids and nutritional supplements. • Blood transfusions may be needed. • Plasmapheresis is sometimes used to remove antibodies from the blood. • Protein limitation and ACE inhibitors to prevent permanent kidney damage.

Mortality rates are 3-5%, but chronic renal problems develop in 50% and a few have lifelong complications, including blindness, paralysis, and kidney failure requiring dialysis.

Multi-Organ Dysfunction Syndrome

Multi-organ dysfunction syndrome is progressive deterioration and failure of 2 or more organ systems with mortality rates of 45-50% with 2 organ systems involved and up to 80-100% if there are ≥3 systems failing. Trauma patients and those with severe conditions, such as shock, burns, and sepsis, are particularly vulnerable. In children, MODS is frequently associated with sepsis, septic shock, or SIRS.

MODS may be primary or secondary:
- Primary MODS relates to direct injury/disorder of the organ systems, resulting in dysfunction, such as with thermal injuries, traumatic pulmonary injuries, and invasive infections.
- Secondary MODS relates to dysfunction of organ systems not directly involved in injury/disorder but developing as the result of a systemic inflammatory response syndrome (SIRS) as the patient's immune and inflammatory responses become dysregulated. In some patients, failure of organ systems is sequential, usually progressing from the lungs, the liver, the gastrointestinal system, and the kidneys to the heart. However, in other cases, various organ systems may fail at the same time.

Multi-System Trauma

Multi-system trauma is very common in children because of their small size and lack of protective musculature to protect internal organs. Because the rib cage and skull are relatively elastic, severe internal injuries can result without external evidence, such as fractures:
- Primary assessment includes establishing patent airway and determining if there is hemorrhage or other compromise of circulation. A neurological survey to determine if there are alterations in consciousness or neurological responses must be done. The child's entire body should be examined for signs of injury. The child's condition should be stabilized and any injuries treated as appropriate (assessment, interventions, and reassessment).
- Secondary assessment includes reassessment of all identified injuries as well as a complete history and physical exam to determine if there are other injuries. If child abuse is expected, determining if the history and presentation of injuries is consistent is important, as are follow-up radiographs to examine for old injuries.

Multisystem Complications Of Burn Injuries

Cardiovascular and Pulmonary
Burn injuries begin with the skin but can affect all organs and body systems, especially with a major burn:
- Cardiovascular: Cardiac output may fall by 50% as capillary permeability increases with vasodilation and fluid leaks from the tissues.
- Urinary: Decreased blood flow causes kidneys to increase ADH, which increases oliguria. BUN and creatinine levels increase. Cell destruction may block tubules, and hematuria may result from hemolysis.

- Pulmonary: Injury may result from smoke inhalation or (rarely) aspiration of hot liquid. Pulmonary injury is a leading cause of death from burns and is classified according to degree of damage:
  1. First: Singed eyebrows and nasal hairs with possible soot in airways and slight edema.
  2. Second: (At 24 hours) Stridor, dyspnea, and tachypnea with edema and erythema of upper airway, including area of vocal chords and epiglottis.
  3. Third: (At 72 hours) worsening symptoms if not intubated and if intubated, bronchorrhea and tachypnea with edematous, secreting tissue.

Neurological, GI, Endocrine/Metabolic

Multisystem complications of burn injuries include:
- Neurological: Encephalopathy may develop from lack of oxygen, decreased blood volume and sepsis. Hallucinations, alterations in consciousness, seizures and coma may result for recovery is usual.
- Gastrointestinal: Ileus and ulcerations of mucosa often result from poor circulation. Ileus usually clears within 48-72 hours, but if it returns it is often indicative of sepsis.
- Endocrine/Metabolic: The sympathetic nervous system stimulates the adrenals to release epinephrine and norepinephrine to increase cardiac output and cortisol for wound healing. The metabolic rate increases markedly. Electrolyte loss occurs with fluid loss from exposed tissue, especially phosphorus, calcium and sodium, with an increase in potassium levels. Electrolyte imbalance can be life-threatening if burns cover >20% of BSA. Glycogen depletion occurs within 12-24 hours and protein breakdown and muscle wasting occurs without sufficient intake of protein.

Management Of Burn Injuries

Management of burn injuries must include both wound care and systemic care to avoid complications that can be life threatening.

Treatment includes:

Establishment of airway and treatment for inhalation injury as indicated:
- Supplemental oxygen, incentive spirometry, nasotracheal suctioning.
- Humidification.
- Bronchoscopy as needed to evaluate bronchospasm and edema.
- β-Agonists for bronchospasm, followed by aminophylline if ineffective.
- Intubation and ventilation if there are indications of respiratory failure. This should be done prior to failure. Tracheostomy may be done if ventilation >14 days.

Intravenous fluids and electrolytes, based on weight of child and extent of burn. Parkland formula: 4 ml/kg/wt x BSA per 24 hours.

Enteral feedings, usually with small lumen feeding tube into the duodenum.

NG tube for gastric decompression to prevent aspiration.

Indwelling catheter to monitor urinary output. Urinary output should be 0.5-2 ml/kg/hr.

Analgesia for reduction of pain and anxiety.

Topical and systemic antibiotics.
Wound care with removal of eschar and dressings as indicated.

Near drowning

Laryngospasm Vs Aspiration
Near-drowning is a common cause of accidents in children, especially in swimming pools, but in adolescents and adults, the incidents most commonly occur in lakes, rivers, and oceans and are related to risk-taking, or altered level of awareness because of drugs or alcohol. Submersion usually causes aspiration (wet drowning) but may trigger severe laryngospasm (dry drowning):

Laryngospasm sequence	Aspiration sequence
• Cardiac arrest with hypoxic/acidosis to brain. • Decreased oxygen, glucose, and adenosine triphosphate. • Decreased sodium, potassium pump. • Increased Na and water in intracranial fluid. • Cerebral intracellular edema leading to neuronal death.	• Cardiac arrest with hypoxic/acidosis to other organs (heart, kidneys). • Decreased oxygen, glucose, adenosine triphosphate. • Decreased sodium, potassium pump. • Increased Na and water in intracranial fluid. • Hypovolemia with shock and death.

Submersion Asphyxia
Sumersion asphyxiation can cause profound damage to the central nervous system, pulmonary dysfunction related to aspiration; cardiac hypoxia with life-threatening arrhythmias, fluid and electrolyte imbalances, and multi-organ damage, so treatment can be complex. Hypothermia related to near drowning has some protective affect because blood is shunted to the brain and heart.

Treatment includes:
- Immediate establishment of airway, breathing and circulation (ABCs).
- High flow 100% oxygen with face mask with intubation if respiratory distress worsens.
- NG tube and decompression to reduce risk of aspiration.
- Fluid management to prevent/ control cerebral/pulmonary edema.
- Neurological evaluation.
- Pulmonary management includes monitoring for ≥72 hours for respiratory deterioration. Ventilation may need positive-end expiratory pressure (PEEP), but this poses danger to cardiac output and can cause barotrauma, so use should be limited.
- Monitoring of cardiac output and function.
- Neurological care to reduce cerebral edema and increased intracranial pressure, and prevent secondary injury.
- Treat GI stress ulcers and acute renal failure.

Continuum of Severe Infections

<u>Bacteremia, Septicemia, Systemic Inflammatory Response Syndrome</u>
There are a number of terms used to refer to severe infections and often used interchangeably, but they are part of a continuum:
- Bacteremia is the present of bacteria in the blood but without systemic infection.
- Septicemia is a systemic infection caused by pathogens (usually bacteria or fungi) present in the blood.
- Systemic inflammatory response syndrome (SIRS), a generalized inflammatory response affecting may organ systems, may be caused by infectious or non-infectious agents, such as trauma, burns, adrenal insufficiency, pulmonary embolism, and drug overdose. If an infectious agent is identified or suspected, SIRS is an aspect of sepsis. Infective agents for children include a wide range of bacteria and fungi, including *Streptococcus pneumoniae* and *Staphylococcus aureus*. SIRS includes 2 of the following:
  - Elevated (>38°C) or subnormal rectal temperature (<36°C)
  - Tachypnea >60 for infants or >50 for children or $PaCO_2$ <32 mm Hg.
  - Tachycardia >160 for infants or >150 for children.
  - Leukocytosis (>12,000) or leukopenia (<4000).

<u>Sepsis, Severe Sepsis, Septic Shock, and MODS</u>
In additions to bacteremia, septicemia, and SIRS, the continuum of severe infections includes:
- Sepsis is presence of infection either locally or systemically in which there is a generalized life-threatening inflammatory response (SIRS). It includes all the indications for SIRS as well as one of the following:
  - Changes in mental status.
  - Hypoxemia (<72 mm Hg) without pulmonary disease.
  - Elevation in plasma lactate.
  - Decreased urinary output <5 ml/kg/wt for ≥1 hour.
- Severe sepsis includes both indications of SIRS and sepsis as well as indications of increasing organ dysfunction with inadequate perfusion and/or hypotension.
- Septic shock is a progression from severe sepsis in which refractory hypotension occurs despite treatment. There may be indications of lactic acidosis.
- Multi-organ dysfunction syndrome (MODS) is the most common cause of sepsis-related death. Cardiac function becomes depressed, acute respiratory distress syndrome (ARDS) may develop, and renal failure may follow acute tubular necrosis or cortical necrosis. Thrombocytopenia appears in about 30% of those affected and may result in disseminated intravascular coagulation (DIC). Liver damage and bowel necrosis may occur.

Septic shock

<u>Symptoms</u>
Septic shock is caused by toxins produced by bacteria and cytokines that the body produces in response to severe infection, resulting in a complex syndrome of disorders.

Symptoms are wide-ranging:
- Initial: Hyper- or hypothermia, increased temperature (>38ºC) with chills, tachycardia with increased pulse pressure, tachypnea, alterations in mental status (dullness), hypotension, hyperventilation with respiratory alkalosis (PaCO$_2$ ≤30 mm Hg), increased lactic acid, and unstable BP, and dehydration with increased urinary output.
- Cardiovascular: Myocardial depression and dysrhythmias.
- Respiratory: Tachypnea, respiratory failure and hypoxia.
- Renal: Acute renal failure (ARF) with ↓urinary output and ↑BUN.
- Hepatic: Jaundice and liver dysfunction with ↑in transaminase, alkaline phosphatase and bilirubin.
- Hematologic: Mild or severe blood loss (from mucosal ulcerations), neutropenia or neutrophilia, decreased platelets, and DIC.
- Endocrine: Hyperglycemia, hypoglycemia (rare).
- Skin: cellulitis, erysipelas, and fascitis, acrocyanotic and necrotic peripheral lesions.

Diagnosis and Treatment
Septic shock is most common in newborns, those >50, and those who are immunocompromised. There is no specific test to confirm a diagnosis of septic shock, so diagnosis is based on clinical findings and tests that evaluate hematologic, infectious, and metabolic states: CBC, DIC panel, electrolytes, liver function tests, BUN, creatinine, blood glucose, ABGs, urinalysis, ECG, radiographs, blood and urine cultures.

Treatment must be aggressive and includes:
- Oxygen and endotracheal intubation as necessary.
- IV access with 2-large bore catheters and central venous line.
- Rapid fluid administration of NS at 10 mL/kg to total of 60 mL/kg or isotonic crystalloid every 5-10 minutes
- Monitoring urinary output.
- Inotropic agents (dopamine, dobutamine, norepinephrine) if no response to fluids or fluid overload.
- Empiric IV antibiotic therapy (usually with 2 broad spectrum antibiotics for both gram-positive and gram-negative bacteria) until cultures return and antibiotics may be changed.
- Hemodynamic and laboratory monitoring.
- Removing source of infection (abscess, catheter).

Children Presenting with Toxic Ingestions

Assessment
Pediatric poisoning is one of the most common medical problems with young children, accounting for about 5% of childhood mortality. Over 90% of poisonings occur within the home environment and over half of toxic poisonings occur to children <6. Most poisonings of young children are accidental and involve small amounts of one substance, generally a household product, such as cosmetics, or medications. Adolescent poisoning is more often intentional, as a suicide attempt or substance abuse, often with multiple substances ingested and a delay in treatment. Recreational drugs, such as Ecstasy, have been implicated in increased poisonings.
Assessment of children with suspected ingestion of toxic substances includes:

- **A**irway.
- **B**reathing.
- **C**irculation.
- **D**isability, drugs/decontamination
- **E**CG, exposure.

Thorough examination to determine the *toxidrome* (characteristic patterns of *symptoms* related to specific toxins) must include assessment of the following:
- Vital sign changes.
- Alterations in mental status.
- Specific symptoms.
- Clinical findings.
- Results of laboratory testing, including serum and urine toxicology screens.

<u>Treatment</u>
Treatment for toxic ingestions is related to the type of toxin and whether or not it is identified.

Treatment includes:
- Administering antidote if substance is known and an antidote exists. Antidotes for common toxins include:
  o Opiates: Naloxone (Narcan®)
  o Toxic alcohols: Ethanol infusion and/or dialysis.
  o Acetaminophen: N-acetylcysteine.
  o Calcium channel blockers, beta-blockers: Calcium chloride, Glucagon.
  o Tricyclic antidepressants: Sodium bicarbonate.
- GI decontamination at one time was standard procedures (Ipecac® and gastric lavage followed by activated charcoal), It is no longer advised for routine use although selective gastric lavage may be appropriate if done within 1 hour of ingestion.
- Activated charcoal (1 g/kg/wt) orally or per NG tube binds to many toxins if given within one hour of ingestion. It may also be used in multiple doses (q 4-6 hrs) to enhance elimination
- Forced diuresis with alkalinization of urine (>7.5) may prevent absorption of drugs that are weak bases or acids.

Acetaminophen toxicity

Acetaminophen toxicity from accidental or intentional overdose has high rates of morbidity and mortality unless promptly treated. Diagnosis is by history and acetaminophen level, which should be completed within 8 hours of ingestion if possible. Toxicity is plotted on the Rumack-Matthew nomogram with serum levels ↑150 requiring antidote. Toxicity occurs with dosage >140 mg/kg in one dose or >7.5g in 24 hours.

Symptoms
- (Initial) Minor gastrointestinal upset.
- (Days 2-3) Hepatotoxicity with RUQ pain and increased AST, ALT, and bilirubin.
- (Days 3-4) Hepatic failure with metabolic acidosis, coagulopathy, renal failure, encephalopathy, nausea, vomiting, and possible death.

- (Days 5-12) Recovery period for survivors.

Treatment
- GI decontamination with activated charcoal (orally or NG) within ≤4 hours.
- Gastric lavage if within 1 hour (may not be effective in small children because of size of NG tube).
- Antidote: 72-hour N-acetylcysteine (NAC) protocol includes 140 mg/kg initially and 70 mg/kg every 4 hours for 17 more doses (orally or IV). Children >40 kg IV administration of 150mg/kg over 1 hour, diluted in 500 mL D% followed by maintenance dose of 100 mg/kg over 16 hours in 1000 mL D5W
- Supportive therapy.

(The antidote is most effective ≤8 hours of ingestion but decreases hepatotoxicity even >24 hours.)

Caustic Ingestions

Caustic ingestions of acids (pH <7) such as sulfuric, acetic, hydrochloric, and hydrofluoric found in many cleaning agents and alkalis (pH >7) such as sodium hydroxide, potassium hydroxide, sodium tripolyphosphate (in detergents) and sodium hypochlorite (bleach) can result in severe injury and death. Acids cause coagulation necrosis in the esophagus and stomach and may result in metabolic acidosis, hemolysis, and renal failure if systemically absorbed. Alkali injuries cause liquefaction necrosis, resulting in deeper ulcerations, often of the esophagus, but may involve perforation and abdominal necrosis with multi-organ damage. *Symptoms* vary but include pain, dyspnea, oral burns, dysphonia, and vomiting. *Diagnosis:* detailed history, airway examination (oral intubation if possible), arterial blood gas, electrolytes, CBC, hepatic and coagulation tests, and radiograph, CT for perforations.

Treatment includes:
- Supportive and symptomatic therapy.
- NO ipecac, charcoal, neutralization, or dilution.
- NG tube for acids only to aspirate residual.
- Endoscopy in first few hours to evaluate injury/perforations.
- Sodium bicarbonate for pH <7.10.
- Prednisolone (alkali injuries).

Amphetamine and Cocaine Toxicity

Amphetamine toxicity may be caused by IV, inhalation, or insufflation of various substances that include methamphetamine (MDA or "ecstasy"), methylphenidate (Ritalin®), methylenedio-xymethamphetamine (MDMA), and ephedrine and phenylpro-panolamine.

Cocaine may be ingested orally, IV or by insufflation while crack cocaine may be smoked. Amphetamines and cocaine are CNS stimulants that can cause multi-system abnormalities. Symptoms may include chest pain, dysrhythmias, myocardial ischemia, MI, seizures, intracranial infarctions, hypertension, dystonia, repetitive movements, unilateral blindness, lethargy, rhabdomyolysis with acute kidney failure, perforated nasal septum (cocaine) and paranoid psychosis (amphetamines).

Crack cocaine may cause pulmonary hemorrhage, asthma, pulmonary edema, barotrauma, and pneumothorax. Swallowing packs of cocaine can cause intestinal ischemia, colitis, necrosis, and perforation. Diagnosis includes clinical findings, CBC, chemistry panel, toxicology screening, ECG, and radiography.

Treatment includes:
- Gastric emptying (≤1 hour).
- Charcoal administration.
- IV access.
- Supplemental oxygen.
- Sedation for seizures: Lorazepam 2m, diazepam 5mg IV titrated in repeated doses.
- Agitation: Haloperidol.
- Hypertension: Nitroprusside, phentolamine 2.5-5mg IV.
- Cocaine quinidine-like effects: Sodium bicarbonate.

Gastric Emptying

Gastric emptying for toxic substance ingestion should be done ≤60 minutes of ingestion for large life-threatening amounts of poison. The patient requires IV access, oximetry, and cardiac monitoring. Sedation (1-2 mg IV midazolam) or RSI and endotracheal intubation may be necessary. Patients should be positioned in left latera decubitus position with head down at 20º to prevent passage of stomach contents into duodenum although intubated patients may be lavaged in the supine position. With a bite block in place, an orogastric Y-tube (24-28 Fr. for children) should be inserted after estimating length. Placement should be confirmed with injection of up to 50 mL of air confirmed under auscultation and aspiration of gastric contents. Irrigation is done by gravity instillation of 10mL/kg warmed (45º C) NS. The instillation side is clamped and drainage side opened. This is repeated until fluid returns clear. A slurry of charcoal is then instilled, and tube clamped and removed when procedures completed.

Carbon Monoxide Poisoning
Carbon monoxide (CO) poisoning occurs with inhalation of fossil fuel exhausts from engines, emission of gas or coal heaters, indoor use of charcoal, and smoke and fumes. The OC binds with hemoglobin, preventing oxygen carriage and impairing oxygen delivery to tissue. *Diagnosis* includes history, on-site oximetry reports, neurological examination, and CO neuropsychological screening battery (CONSB) done with patient breathing room air, CBC, electrolytes, ABGs, ECG, chest radiograph (for dyspnea).

Symptoms	Treatment
• Cardiac: chest pain, palpitations, ↓ capillary refill, hypotension, cardiac arrest. • CNS: malaise, nausea, vomiting, lethargy, stroke, coma, seizure. • Secondary injuries: rhabdomyolysis with renal failure • Non-cardiogenic pulmonary edema • Multiple organs failure (MOF). • DIC. • Encephalopathy.	• Immediate support of airway, breathing, and circulation. • Non-barometric oxygen (100%) by non-breathing mask with reservoir or ETT if necessary. • Mild: Continue oxygen for 4 hours with reassessment. • Severe: hyperbaric oxygen therapy (usually 3 treatments) to improve oxygen delivery.

Cyanide Poisoning

Cyanide poisoning, from hydrogen cyanide (HCN) or cyanide salts, can result from inhalation of burning plastics, intentional or accidental ingestion or dermal exposure, occupation exposure, ingestion of some plant products, manufacture of PCP, and sodium nitroprusside infusions. Inhalation of HCN causes immediate symptoms; and ingestion of cyanide salts, within minutes. *Diagnosis* is by history, clinical examination, and normal PaO_2 and metabolic acidosis. *Symptoms* increase in severity and alter with the amount of exposure:

Symptoms	Treatment

• **Cardiovascular**: tachycardia, hypertension, bradycardia, hypotension, and cardiac arrest.
• **Skin**: May appear pink or cherry-colored because of oxygen remaining in the blood.
• **CNS**: Headaches, lethargy, seizures, coma.
• **Respiratory**: Dyspnea, tachypnea, and respiratory arrest.
	• Supportive care as indicated.
	• Removal of contaminated clothes.
	• Gastric decontamination.
	• Copious irrigation for topical exposure.
	• Antidotes:
	  o Amyl nitrate ampule cracked and inhaled 30 seconds.
	  o Sodium nitrite (3%) 10 mL IV.
	  o Sodium thiosulfate (25%) 50 mL IV.
	(Children's doses of sodium nitrite and sodium thiosulfate adjusted according to hemoglobin level.)

Salicylate Toxicity

Salicylate toxicity may be acute or chronic and is caused by ingestion of OTC drugs containing salicylates, such as ASA, Pepto-Bismol®, and products used in hot inhalers. Diagnosis is by ferric chloride or Ames Phenytex tests. Symptoms vary according to age and amount of ingestion, and co-ingestion of sedatives may alter symptoms.

Symptoms	Treatment
• <150 mg/kg: nausea and vomiting. • 150-300 mg/kg: Vomiting, hyperpnea, diaphoresis, tinnitus, and alterations in acid-base balance. • >300 mg/kg: Metabolic acidosis in children <4 but respiratory alkalosis and metabolic acidosis with alkalemia (pH >7.5) in older children. Chronic toxicity is more serious and includes hyperventilation, volume depletion, acidosis, hypokalemia, and CNS abnormalities.	• Gastric decontamination with lavage ($\leq$1 hour) and charcoal. • Volume replacement (D5W). • Sodium bicarbonate 1-2mEq/kg. • Monitoring of salicylate concentration, acid-base, and electrolytes every hour. • Whole-bowel irrigation (sustained release tablets).

Benzodiazepine Toxicity

Benzodiazepine toxicity may result from accidental or intentional overdose with such drugs as Xanax®, Librium®, Valium®, Ativan®, Serax®, Versed®, and Restoril®. Mortality is usually the result of co-ingestion of other drugs. Diagnosis is based on history and clinical exam, as benzodiazepine level does not correlate well with toxicity.

Symptoms	Treatment
• Non-specific neurological changes: lethargy, dizziness, alterations in consciousness, ataxia. • Respiratory depression and hypotension are rare complications. • Coma and severe central nervous depression are usually caused by co-ingestions.	• Gastric emptying (<1 hour). • Charcoal. • Concentrated dextrose, thiamine and naloxone if co-ingestions suspected, especially with altered mental status. • Monitoring for CNS/respiratory depression. • Supportive care. • Flumazenil (antagonist) 0.2mg each minute to total 3mg may be used in some cases but not routinely advised because of complications related to benzodiazepine dependency or co-ingestion of cyclic antidepressants. Flumazenil is contraindicated in the presence of increased intracranial pressure.

Ethanol Overdose

Ethanol overdose affects the central nervous system as well as other organs in the body. Ethanol is absorbed through the mucosa of the mouth, stomach, and intestines, with concentrations peaking in about 30-60 minutes. Young children often ingest alcohol in products (perfumes, cleaning solutions) that are more toxic than alcoholic beverages. The liver clears ethanol more rapidly than in adults, at about 30 mg/dL/hr or about 0.5 ounce/hr.

Symptoms	Treatment
Infants/young children: Seizures and coma. Respiratory depression and hypoxia. Hypoglycemia (especially infants and toddlers). Hypothermia. **Adolescents:** Altered mental status. Hypotension. Bradycardia with arrhythmias Respiratory depression and hypoxia. Cold, clammy skin or flushed skin (from vasodilation). Acute pancreatitis with abdominal pain. Lack of consciousness. Circulatory collapse, death.	Monitor of arterial blood gases and oxygen saturation. Ensure patent airway with intubation and ventilation if necessary. Intravenous fluids. Dextrose to correct hypoglycemia. Maintain body temperature (warming blanket). Dialysis in severe cases.

Pain Assessment of Neonates/Infants

Pain assessment of neonates and infants depends on careful obser-vation of a number of characteristics. The Neonate/infant Pain Scale (NIPS) assesses 6 areas with a score >3 indicating pain. Five areas are scored 0-1, depending upon the degree of stress. Crying, which is often the most indicative of pain, is scored 0-2:

Character-istic	0	1	2
Expression on face	Rested, normal	Negative, tightened muscles, grimace	
Crying	None	Intermittent, moaning, whimper	Loud, shrill continuous crying
Respira-tory patterns	Relaxed, normal	Changes include irregular breathing, tachypnea, holding breath, gagging	
Upper ex-tremeities	Relaxed, ran-dom movement	Tense, rigid or rapid extending and flexing.	
Lower ex-tremeities	Relaxed, ran-dom movement	Tense, rigid or rapid extending and flexing.	
Arousal state	Quiet, awake or asleep with random leg movements	Restless, fussing, thrashing about.	

Pain Assessment of Children 1-7

The Children's Hospital Eastern Ontario Pain Scale (CHEOPS) is used for children 1-7 and is based on scores of 6 different characteristics with scores of 0-2 except for crying, which is scored 0-3. A score >4 indicate pain.

Crying
1 - Not crying
2 -Silent crying, moaning, or whimpering
3 - Sobbing, screaming

Facial expression
0-Smiling, positive
1 – Neutral
2- Grimacing, negative

Verbalization
0- Positive, no complaints
1- 1 - Not talking or complaining about other things (not pain).
2- 2 -Complaining about pain or pain and other things.

Torso
1- Inactive, at rest, relaxed
2 - Tense, moving, shuddering, shivering, and/or sitting upright or restrained.

Upper extremities
1 - Not touching or reaching for wound or injury.
2 - Reaching for, touching gently, or grabbing wound or injury or arms restrained.

Lower extremities
1 - Relaxed, random movement.
2 - Restless or tense moving or legs flexed, kicking crouching, kneeling, or legs restrained.

Note: Children over 7 may be able to describe pain or indicate pain according to facial expression scale, but this may be difficult for younger children.

Pre-Teen/Adolescent Pain Scale

Pain is subjective and may be influenced by the individual's pain sensation threshold (the smallest stimulus that produces the sensation of pain) and tolerance threshold (the maximum degree of pain that a person can tolerate). The most common current pain assessment tool for pre-teens and adolescents is the 1-10 pain scale:
- 0 = no pain.
- 1-2 = mild pain.
- 3-5 = moderate pain.
- 6-7 = severe pain.
- 8-9 = very severe pain.
- 10 = excruciating pain.

However, assessment also includes information about onset, duration, and intensity. Identifying pain triggers and what relieves it is essential when developing a pain management plan. Children may show very different behaviors when they are in pain: Some may cry and moan with minor pain, and others may seem indifferent even when they are truly suffering. Thus, judging pain by behavior alone can lead to the wrong conclusions.

Pain Assessment for theCognitively Impaired

The Non-communicating Children's Pain Checklist (NCCPC) is designed for children 3 to 8 who are cognitively impaired but may be used for children recovering from anesthesia (modified version). The checklist contains 7 categories with subllistings that are each scored: 0 (not occuring), 1 occuring occasionally, 2 occurring fairly often, 3 occuring frequently, and NA (not applicable).

Vocal · Moaning, whining · Crying · Screaming, yelling · Specific word for pain

Social · Uncooperative unhappy · Withdrawn · Seeking closeness · Inability to distract

Facial · Furrowed brow · Eye changes · Non-smiling · Lips tight/quivering · Clenching grinding teeth

Activity ·Not moving, quiet · Agitated, fidgety

Body/limbs · Floppy · Tense, rigid, spastic · Pointing to part of body that hurts.   ·
Guarding part of body · Flinching · Positioning body to show pain

Physiological ·Shivering · Pallor · Increased perspiration · Tears · Gasping · Holding
breath

Eating, sleeping ·Eating less · Increased sleep · Decreased sleep

Total scores

The child is usually observed for 2 hours and then scored and all scores added. A score of
≥7 indicates pain.

Equianalgesia

Equianalgesia is a comparison of doses of different analgesics that provide equivalent
analgesia/sedation. Children may vary in their ability to metabolize drugs, so they must be
monitored carefully with all analgesics. Intravenous analgesics usually take effect within 15
to 30 minutes while oral medications take twice as long. Dosage must be calculated
according to age and weight:

Drug	Parenteral	Oral
Morphine sulfate	10 mg (Infants start at 0.05 mg/kg & children at 0.1 mg/kg)	30 mg (Children's dosages vary according to preparation)
Dilaudid	1.5mg (Infants & children start at 0.015 mg/kg)	7.5 mg (Children's dosages vary according to preparation)
Fentanyl	100 mcg (Infants and children start at 0.5 to 2 mcg/kg)	Varies (patches)
Demerol	75 to 100 mg (Infants and children start at 1 to 1.5 mg/kg)	300 mg (Not recommended for children) (Used for shivering but not for analgesia)
Codeine	120 mg (Not recom-mended for children)	200 mg (Children's dosages vary according to preparation).
Vicodin	--	30 mg (Children's dosages vary according to preparation)

Pain Management

Acetaminophen
Dosages may be repeated every 4 hours to maximum of 5 in 24 hours. Dosage based on 10
to 15 mg/kg with adult dosing at 12 years:
- 0 to 3 months: 40 mg (to maximum of 200/24 hr).
- 2 to 3 years: 120 mg (to maximum of 600 mg/24 hr.)
- 6 to 8 years: 320 mg (to maximum of 1600 mg/24 hr.)
- 11 years: 480mg (to maximum of 2400/24 hr.)

Side Effects:
Allergic response with itching, rash, edema.
Liver toxicity with overdose.

Choline magnesium trisalicylate
- <37 kg/81.5 lb: 50 mg/kg/d divided in 2 doses.
- >37 kg/81.5 lb: 2250 mg/d divided in 2 doses.

Side Effects:
Tinnitus. GI irritation with nausea, vomiting, diarrhea, constipation, epigastric discomfort.

Ibuprofen
- <6 months to 12 years: 5 to 10 mg/kg every 6 to 8 hours (to maximum of 40 mg/kg/day).
- 12 to 18 years: 200 to 400 mg every 4 to 6 hours to maximum of 2400 mg/day.

Side Effects:
Nausea, vomiting, diarrhea. Gastrointestinal irritation with ulcerations and bleeding. Bleeding nephritis. Retention of fluid.

Naprosyn
>2 years: 20 mg/kg/day divided in 2 doses.

Side Effects:
Same as ibuprofen.

Tolmetin
>2 years: 20 g/kg/day divided in 3 to 4 doses.

Side Effects:
Same as ibuprofen.

Patient-Controlled Analgesia

Patient-controlled analgesia (PCA) allows the child to control administration of pain medication by pressing a button on an intravenous delivery system with a computerized pump. The device is filled with opioid (as prescribed) and must be programmed correctly and checked regularly to ensure that it is functioning properly and that controls are set. The most-commonly administered medications include morphine, meperidine, fentanyl, and sufentanil. Most devices can be set to deliver continuous infusion of opioid as well as patient-controlled bolus.

Each element must be set:
- Bolus: Determines the amount of medication received when the patient delivers a dose.
- Lockout interval: Time required between administrations of boluses.
- Continuous infusion: Rate at which opioid is delivered per hour for continuous analgesia.

- Limit (usually set at 4 hours): Total amount of opioid that can be delivered in the preset time limit.

With Authorized Agent Controlled Analgesia (AACA), people who are trained and authorized (such as nurse, family member, and caregiver) may administer the medication as well as the child.

Non-pharmacologic Pain Management

Non-pharmacologic Methods of Managing Pain	
Behavioral contracting	Use rewards (stickers, privileges) for compliance and cooperation, Write up contract that outlines expectations and rewards for compliance and cooperation (such as not hitting during dressing changes).
Distraction	Encourage games, radio, TV, play, music, deep breathing, blowing bubbles, and reading books.
Guided imagery	Encourage child to think of a pleasant event and describe it, concentrating on all aspects of the event (sounds, feelings, tastes, colors, smells).
Positive thinking	Teach child to make positive statements: "I will feel better soon." Teach child to counter focus on negative experiences with positive thoughts: "The shot only lasts a few seconds."
Relaxation exercises	Infant, small child: Hold and rock or sway back and forth. Older child: Use progressive relaxation by tightening and relaxing parts of body.

Therapeutic Hypothermia

Therapeutic hypothermia is used to reduce ischemic tissue damage associated with cardiac arrest, ischemic stroke, traumatic brain/spinal cord injury, neurogenic fever, and related coma (3 on Glasgow scale). Hypothermia has a neuroprotective effect by making cell membranes less permeable. Hypothermia should be initiated immediately after an ischemic event if possible but some benefit remains up to 6 hours. Desflurane or meperidine is given to reduce the shivering response. Hypothermia to 33°C may be induced by cooled saline through a femoral catheter, reducing temperature 1.5 to 2° C per hour, with by an electronic control unit. Hypothermic water blankets covering ≥80% of body the body surface can also lower body temperature. In some cases, both a femoral cooling catheter and water blanket are used for rapid reduction of temperature. Rectal probes measure core temperature. Hypothermia increases risk of bleeding (decreased clotting time), infection (from catheter), and DVT. Rewarming is done slowly at 0.5 to 1° C/hr. through warmed intravenous fluids, warm humidified air, and/or warming blanket.

Conscious Sedation

Conscious sedation is used to decrease sensations of pain and awareness caused by a surgical or invasive procedure, such a biopsy, chest tube insertion, fracture repair, and endoscopy. It is also used during presurgical preparations, such as insertion of central lines, catheters, and use of cooling blankets. Conscious sedation uses a combination of analgesia and sedation so that patients can remain responsive and follow verbal cues but have a brief amnesia preventing recall of the procedures. The patient must be monitored carefully, including pulse oximetry, during this type of sedation. The most commonly used drugs include:

- Midazolam (Versed®): This is a short-acting water-soluble sedative, with onset of 1-5 minutes, peaking in 30, and duration usually about 1 hour (but may last up to 6 hours).
- Fentanyl: This is a short-acting opioid with immediate onset, peaking in 10-15 minutes and with duration of about 20-45 minutes.

The fentanyl/midazolam combination provides both sedation and pain control. Conscious sedation usually requires 6 hours fasting prior to administration.

Postoperative Nausea and Vomiting

Post-operative nausea and vomiting (PONV) varies with the type of anesthetic agent used. It occurs in about 20-30% of post-anesthesia patients and may be delayed up to 24 hours. Inhalational agents have a higher incidence of PONV than intravenous, and the incidence is lower with epidural or subarachnoid administration although it may indicate the onset of hypotension. PONV correlates with the duration of surgery, with longer surgeries causing increased PONV. If high doses of narcotics, propofol, or nitrous oxide are used, PONV is often a problem. PONV is most common in young females and also relates to menstruation. It is also increased in those with a history of smoking or motion sickness. Some surgical procedures correlate with PONV: strabismus repair, ear surgery, laparoscopy, tonsillectomy, orchiopexy, and gynecological procedures to retrieve ova. PONV may be associated with post-operative pain, so managing pain is an important factor in preventing PONV.

Post-Anesthetic Complications

Respiratory

Respiratory complications are the most common in the postanesthesia period, so monitoring of oxygen levels is critical to preventing hypoxemia:

- Airway obstruction may be partial or total. Partial obstruction is indicated by sonorous or wheezing respirations, and total by absence of breath sounds. Treatment includes supplemental oxygen, airway insertion, repositioning (jaw thrust), or succinylcholine and positive-pressure ventilation for laryngospasm. If edema of the glottis is causing obstruction, IV corticosteroids may be used.
- Hypoventilation ($PaCO_2$ >45 mm Hg) is often mild but may cause respiratory acidosis. It is usually related to depression caused by anesthetic agents. A number of factors may slow emergence (hypothermia, overdose, metabolism) and cause hypoventilation. It may also be related to splinting because of pain, requiring additional pain management.
- Hypoxemia (mild is PaO_2 500-60 mm Hg) is usually related to hypoventilation and/or increased right to left shunting and is usually treated with supplementary oxygen (30-60%) with or without positive airway pressure.

Cardiovascular

Cardiovascular complications are sometimes related to respiratory complications, which may need to be addressed as well. Complications include:

- Hypotension is most often mild and requires no specific treatment. It is most commonly caused by hypovolemia and is significant if BP falls 20-30% below normal baseline. A bolus of IV colloid is used to confirm hypovolemia. If severe, then medications, such as epinephrine, may be indicated. Hypotension may occur with pneumothorax so careful respiratory assessment must be done.
- Hypertension usually occurs ≤ 30 minutes after surgery and is common in those with history of hypertension. It may be secondary to hypoxemia or metabolic acidosis. Mild increases usually don't require treatment but medications may be used for moderate (β-adrenergic blockers) or severe (nitroprusside).
- Arrhythmias usually relate to respiratory complications or effects of anesthetic agents. Bradycardia may relate to cholinesterase inhibitors, opioids, or propranolol. Tachycardia may relate to anticholinergics, β-agonists, and vagolytic drugs. Hypokalemia and hypomagnesemia may cause premature atrial and ventricular beats.

Behavioral/Psychosocial

Child Abuse

Reporting Requirements

About 5 million cases of suspected child abuse are reported in the United States each year. In accordance with the Child Abuse Prevention and Treatment and Adoption Act Amendments (1996) and the Model Child Protection Act, all states have instituted mandatory reporting of child abuse. The nurse should be knowledgeable about the statutes in the state of practice, but medical personnel are mandatory reporters and must report the following:
- Child abuse or neglect that places the child in risk of harm (physical or emotional), death, or exploitation.
- Sexual abuse including rape, molestation, prostitution, incest, or engaging in any type of sexually explicit behavior.

While some statutes mandate reporting mere suspicion, others mandate only reporting specific knowledge. Regardless, there is criminal and civil liability involved if child abuse is not reported, and most states provide immunity for reporters. Thus, the best course is to report even suspicions to child protective services or the police, according to the state requirements.

Physical and Behavioral Signs

Children rarely admit to abuse and, in fact, typically deny it and attempt to protect the abusing parent. Therefore, the critical care nurse must often rely on physical and behavioral signs to determine if there is cause to suspect abuse:
- Behavioral indicators: The child may be overly compliant or fearful with obvious changes in demeanor when a parent/caregiver is present. Some children act out with aggression toward other children or animals. Children may become depressed or suicidal or present with sleeping or eating disorders. Behaviors may become increasingly self-destructive as the child ages, including inappropriate sexualized behavior.
- Physical indicators: The type, location, and extent of injuries can raise suspicion of abuse. Head and facial injuries and bruising are common, as are bite or burn marks. There may be hand prints or grab marks, unusual bruising, such as across the buttocks. Any bruising, swelling, or tearing of the genital area and the identification of sexually transmitted diseases are also causes for concern.

Signs of Neglect and Lack of Supervision

While some children may not be physically or sexually abused, they may suffer from profound neglect or lack of supervision that places them at risk.

Indicators include:
- Appearing dirty and unkempt, sometimes with infestations of lice, and wearing ill fitting, torn clothing and shoes.
- Being tired and sleepy during the daytime.
- Having excessive medical or dental problems, such as extensive dental caries.
- Missing doctor's appointments and not receiving proper immunizations.

- Being underweight for their current stage of development.

Neglect can be difficult to assess, especially if the critical care nurse is serving a homeless or very disadvantaged population. Home visits may be needed to ascertain if there is adequate food, clothing, or supervision, and this may be beyond the scope of care provided by the critical care nurse. Thus, suspicions should be reported so that social workers can arrange a follow-up assessment of the home environment.

Domestic Violence

According to guidelines of the Family Violence Prevention Fund, assessment for domestic violence should be done for all adolescent patients, regardless of background or signs of abuse. While females are the most common victims, there are increasing reports of male victims of domestic violence, both in heterosexual and homosexual relationships. The person doing the assessment should be informed about domestic violence and be aware or risk factors and danger signs. The interview should be conducted in private (or with children <3 years old). The office, bathrooms, and examining rooms should have information about domestic violence posted prominently. Brochures and information should be available to give to patients. Patients may present with a variety of physical complaints, such as headache, pain, palpitations, numbness, or pelvic pain. They are often depressed and may appear suicidal and may be isolated from friends and family. Victims of domestic violence often exhibit fear of perpetrator (such as a parent, boyfriend, or girlfriend) and may report injury inconsistent with symptoms.

Injuries Consistent with Domestic Violence/Abuse

Injuries consistent with domestic violence/abuse	
Characteristic injuries	• Ruptured eardrum. • Rectal/genital injury—burns, bites, trauma. • Scrapes and bruises about the neck, face, head, trunk, arms. • Cuts, bruises, and fractures of the face.
Patterns of injuries	• Bathing suit pattern—injuries on parts of body that are usually covered with clothing as the perpetrator abuses but hides evidence of abuse. • Head and neck injuries (50%).
Abusive injuries (rarely attributable to accidents)	• Bites, bruises, rope and cigarette burns, welts in the outline of weapons (belt marks). • Bilateral injuries of arms/legs.
Defensive injuries	• Back of the body injury from being attacked while crouched on the floor face down. • Soles of the feet from kicking at perpetrator. • Ulnar aspect of hand or palm from blocking blows.

Pervasive Developmental Disorders

Autism
Autism spectrum disorders (ASD), pervasive developmental disorders (PDD), present with a wide range of symptoms. These children, usually exhibiting symptoms within the first 2

- 62 –

years, are often isolated with an inability to socialize. About 25% suffer seizure disorders. Diagnostic criteria include at least 6 of the following:

- Impairment of social interactions (in at least 2 areas): Inability to use/understand non-verbal communication, inability to establish peer relationships, lack of socialization skills, and inability to express emotions.
- Impairment of communication (In at least one area): Delay or lack of spoken language without attempt to compensate, such as through gestures, inability to carry out a conversation with others, repetitive use of language (echolalia), and inability to carry out make-believe play or imitation appropriate to developmental level.
- Restrictive repetitive or stereotyped behavior (in at least one area): Preoccupation with some behavior patterns (head banging, rituals), inflexibility, and/or preoccupation with objects.

Early diagnosis helps maximize the child's potential and may allow the child to live independently as an adult.

Rett's Syndrome

Rett's syndrome is a pervasive developmental disorder in females, characterized by normal prenatal development, normal motor development in the first five months of life and a normal head circumference. However, between 5-48 months of age, head growth decelerates and the loss of purposeful use of the hands, along with gait abnormalities, seizures, and mental retardation appears.

I (Early onset) 6-18 mo. The infant begins to exhibit less eye contact, diminished interest in playing, and delays in motor skill development (crawling and sitting).

II (Rapid destruction) 1-4 yrs. Previously gained skills, such as use of hands and speech, are lost. Purposeless hand movements such as wringing, grasping or finger wriggling begin but disappear when child is asleep. Deceleration of head growth is usually evident.

III (Pseudo-stationary) 2-10 yrs. Apraxia and seizures are prominent. A child may show more interest in her surroundings than she did during Stage II, and her alertness, attention span, and communication skills may improve. Many girls remain in this stage for most of their lives.

IV (Motor deterioration) --- Characterized by reduced mobility, muscle weakness; rigidity spasticity; dystonia and scoliosis are common features. Girls who were previously able to walk may stop walking. Generally, there is no decline in cognition, communi-cation, or hand skills. Repetitive hand movements may decrease, and eye gaze usually improves.

Mental retardation

Mental retardation (MR) is usually diagnosed <18. Individuals may have difficulty adapting to changing environments, need guidance in decision-making, and have self-care or communication deficits. Behaviors range from shy and passive to hyperactive or aggressive. Those with associated physical characteristics (Down syndrome) or problems are often diagnosed early. MR may be inherited (Tay-Sachs), toxin-related (maternal alcohol consumption), perinatal (hypoxia), environmental (lack of stimulation/neglect), or acquired (encephalitis, brain injury). Diagnosis involves performance results from standardized tests along with behavior analysis. MR classifications are based on IQ:

Classifications	Description
55 to 69 – mild (85%):	Educable to about 6th grade level. May not be diagnosed until adolescence. Usually able to learn skills and be self-supporting but may need assistance and supervision.
40 to 54 – moderate 10%):	Trainable and may be able to work and live in sheltered environments or with supervision.
25 to 39 – severe (3-4%):	Language usually delayed and can learn only basic academic skills and perform simple tasks.
≤25 – profound (1-2%):	Usually associated with neurological disorder with sensorimotor dysfunction. Require constant care and supervision.

Failure to Thrive

Failure to thrive (FTT) is a descriptive term for children who exhibit inadequate growth and development, usually measured by the child's being below the 5th percentile for weight (and sometimes height). Failure to thrive may relate to physical causes (such as renal disease or congenital heart disease), psychosocial factors (such as poverty, neglect) or idiopathic factors (unexplained). However, may issues may be involved other than just the parent-child relationship:
- Income: Inability to buy sufficient or nutritional food.
- Health beliefs: Child subjected to extreme or fad diets (Vegan, low fat) without ensuring proper nutrition.
- Lack of education: Inadequate knowledge of proper nutritional requirements for children.
- Stress: Illness, single-family home, divorce, lack of employment, incarceration.
- Psychosocial issues: Post-partum depression, other mental illnesses, or Munchausen syndrome by proxy.
- Resistance to feeding: History of NG feedings, cleft lip/palate, or esophageal atresia,
- Inadequate supply of milk: Poor breastfeeding technique or poor milk supply.

Diagnosis and Management
Failure to thrive (FTT) is diagnosed first by identifying children at risk because of their evidence of growth failure.

Diagnostic measures	Management
Weight/height percentile (5th percentile for weight indicative of FTT). Dietary intake history: Previous 24 hours and 3 to 5 day period. Evaluation of genetic factors: Family history, including heights/weights of parents. Identification of food	Nutritional program to reverse evidence of malnutrition: Formula: Kcal per day = RDA for age in kcal/kg X ideal weight/actual weight. · Vitamin and mineral supplements. · Infants (young): Provide supplements to formula. Kcal per ounce of formula should not exceed 24. · Toddlers: Provide high-

allergies and food restrictions. Evaluation of meal behaviors/ practices. Lab tests as indicated to check for conditions such as anemia, parasites, and lead poisoning. Observation of family interactions, situation.	caloric milk drink (PediaSure). Referrals to social workers, welfare, child protective services as indicated. Behavior modification related to meal times, eating habits interfering with nutrition. Family therapy as indicated. Family education. Structured supportive environment for feeding, Persistence in feeding and elimination of distractions. Slow introduction of new foods.

Use of Restraints

Restraints are used to restrict movement, activity, and access. There are two primary types of restraints used with children, clinical and behavioral. Behavioral restraints are more commonly used in the psychiatric unit or when children are at risk of hurting themselves or others. More commonly, clinical restraints are used to ensure that the child does not interfere with safe care. Restraints may be applied temporarily during a particular treatment or procedure or may be part of permanent care (as with postoperative elbow restraints after cleft lip repair). The Joint Commission has issued strict guidelines for temporary restraints or those not part of standard care (such as post-surgical restraint):
- There must be a written policy.
- An assessment must be completed.
- An alternative method should be tried before applying a restraint.
- An order must be written.
- The least restrictive effective restraint should be used.
- A nurse must remove the restraint, assess, and document findings at least every 2 hours.

Types of Restraints

There are a number of different types of restraints to ensure child safety:
- Swaddling: Used for infants and small children for treatments/ examinations of the head, neck, and throat, venipuncture, and gavage feedings to prevent movement. A papoose board with straps or a mummy wrap is used.
- Jacket: Used to prevent children from falling out of chairs/beds or to maintain horizontal position. A jacket is applied with ties in the back and long ties secured out of reach in the back of the wheelchair or underside of the crib.
- Limb: Used to prevent arm or leg movement that might cause injury or to protect IV access. Commercial restraints are sized, so they should fit properly and should be padded to prevent pressure.
- Elbow: This restraint is used to prevent the child from reaching the head or face, usually after surgery, or to prevent scratching. The most common restraint is a muslin wrap with pockets for tongue depressors for infants. Commercial restraints are available for older children.

Bipolar Disorder

Bipolar disorder causes severe mood swings between hyperactive states and depression, accompanied by impaired judgment because os distorted thoughts. The hypomanic stage may allow for creativity and good functioning in some young people, but it can develop into more severe mania, which may be associated with psychosis and hallucinations, and then into periods of profound depression. While most cases are diagnosed in late adolescents, there is increasing evidence that some children present with symptoms earlier, especially at risk are children's with a bipolar parent. Bipolar disorder is associated with high rates of suicide, so early diagnosis and treatment is critical. Symptoms may be relatively mild or involve severe rapid cycling between mania and depression. Intervention includes both medications (usually given continually) to prevent cycling and control depression and psychosocial therapy, such as cognitive therapy, which helps children control disordered thought patterns and behavior.

Depression

Depression is increasingly recognized as a risk factor for children, manifesting in young children as pretending illness or refusal to go to school and in older children as behavioral problems, negativity, and difficulties at school rather than the more common withdrawal and overt depression of some adults. However, children may feel persistent anxiety and sadness and often have profound fears that something will happen to a parent. Usually changes in behavior become apparent. One study showed that 29% of children with depression had suicidal thoughts, making early diagnosis and intervention very important. While there is some concern about antidepressants and children, suicide is a leading cause of death in teenagers, so medications with careful monitoring along with psychotherapy, such as cognitive behavioral therapy, seem to provide the best form of treatment, providing >70% with clinical improvement.

Eating Disorders

Eating disorders are a profound health risk, especially for young girls although boys sometimes also have eating disorders, often presenting as excessive exercise. Different types include:
- Anorexia nervosa affects 0.5-3.7% of females, characterized by profound fear of weight gain and severe restriction of food intake, often accompanied by abuse of diuretics and laxatives, which can cause electrolyte imbalances as well as kidney and bowel disorders and delay or cessation of menses. Anorexics may become emaciated and risk death.
- Bulimia nervosa affects 1.1-4.2% of females and includes binge eating followed by vomiting often along with diuretics, enemas, and laxatives. Gastric acids can damage the throat and teeth. While bulimics may maintain a normal weight, they are at risk for severe electrolyte imbalances that can be life threatening.
- Binge eating affects 2-5% of females and includes grossly overeating, often resulting in obesity, depression, and shame.

Early intervention can prevent physical damage but may require hospitalization and intense therapy for long periods of time to change altered thinking.

Schizophrenia

Initial Symptoms
Schizophrenia is a psychotic disorder characterized by personality disintegration and distortion in the perception of reality, thought processes and social development with onset usually in late adolescence.

Criteria include:
- Presence of ≥2 of the following for a significant time during a one-month period: delusions, withdrawal, odd behavior, hallucinations, inability to care for self, disorganized speech, catatonia, alogia (inability to speak because of mental deficiency, mental confusion, or aphasia), and avolition (inability to initiate and persist in goal-directed behavior).
- Only one of the above symptoms if the following present:
  o Bizarre delusions such as thought broadcasting or being controlled by a dead person
  o Hearing a voice constantly commenting on a person's behavior or thoughts. The voice may be from God, Satan, a friend or a relative. Individuals experiencing these voices often attempt to quiet or eliminate the voices by turning the radio or television to static to drown out the voices.
  o Hearing two or more voices conversing with each other.
- Social and/or occupational dysfunction for a major portion of time since onset.

Ongoing Symptoms
Schizophrenia is a chronic disorder, so diagnosis requires continuous signs of disturbance for at least six months, including:
- At least one month of active symptoms, *and*
- Prodromal and residual phases that include the following symptoms:
  o Social isolation.
  o Catatonic behavior.
  o Unusual behavior, such as talking to oneself in public.
  o Little attention to personal hygiene.
  o Odd speech characterized by the following:
    ▪ Circumstantiality: Talking in circles around the issue.
    ▪ Tangentiality: Moving from one topic to another where the logical connection may be visible but is not relevant to the issue being discussed.
    ▪ Magical thinking: Including ideas or delusions of reference (such as having magical powers obtained from trees).
    ▪ Recurrent illogical perceptual experiences

Second-Generation/Atypical Antipsychotics

Second-generation antipsychotics (SGAs), also called atypical antipsychotics, are used for bipolar disorders, schizophrenia, and psychosis and include aripiprazole (Abilify®), clozapine (Clozaril®), olanzapine (Zyprexa®), quetiapine (Seroquel®), risperidone (Risperdal®), paliperidone (Invega®), and ziprasidone (Geodon®). Children may also receive atypical antipsychotics for a wide range of non-psychotic disorders, such as mood disorders (most common), eating disorders, developmental disorders (autism spectrum), and tic disorders. Use is most common during adolescence. Children should receive the lowest effective dose of medication.

Side-effects include constipation, increased appetite, weight gain, urinary retention, various sexual side effects, increased prolactin, menstrual irregularities, and increased risk of diabetes mellitus, decreased blood pressure, dizziness, agranulocytosis, and leucopenia. Atypical antipsychotics may interact with fluvoxamine, phenytoin, carbamazepine, barbiturates, nicotine, ketoconazole, phenytoin, rifampin, and glucocorticoids. The use of atypical antipsychotic agents correlates with significant weight gain and suicidal ideation.

Overweight and obese children are likely to develop insulin resistance and glucose intolerance, which may lead to diabetes mellitus.

Selective Serotonin Reuptake Inhibitors

Selective serotonin reuptake inhibitors (SSRIs) are antidepressant medications that block reuptake of serotonin (neurotransmitter) in the brain, increasing the extracellular level of the neurotransmitter and improving transmission. Drugs include citalopram (Celexa®), escitalopram (Lexapro®), fluoxetine (Prozac®), and paroxetine (Paxil). All SSRIs have similar action but may have different chemical properties that cause various side effects, so some children tolerate one better than others. Side effects include nausea, weight gain, sexual dysfunction, excitation and agitation, and insomnia, drowsiness, increased perspiration, headache, and diarrhea. In rare cases, serotonin syndrome may occur from high levels of serotonin from overdose or combination with MAO inhibitors, so SSRIs must not be taken within 2 weeks of each other. Symptoms include severe anxiety and agitation, hallucinations, confusion, blood pressure swings, fever, tachycardia, seizures, and coma. SSRIs are not addictive but abrupt cessation may trigger discontinuation syndrome (flu-like symptoms). Suicidal ideation and increased depression may occur in pediatric patients.

<u>Lithium Carbonate</u>

Lithium carbonate (Eskalith®, Lithobid®) is used to control the manic episodes associated with bipolar disorder. While it is FDA-approved only for children over 12, it is increasingly used for younger children. Children should be started on ≤30mg/kg/day with blood levels monitored every other day initially. Lithium has a very narrow therapeutic window, and toxicity is a medical emergency that can lead to death. Target serum levels are 0.6 to 1.2 mEq/L. Increased blood levels can cause toxicity:

- 1.5 to 2.5 mEq/L: Severe vomiting and diarrhea, increased muscle tremors and twitching, lethargy, body aches, ataxia, ringing in the ears, blurry vision, vertigo or hyperactive deep tendon reflexes.
- >2.5 mEq/L: Elevated temperature, low urine output, hypotension, ECG abnormalities, decreased level of consciousness, seizures, coma or death.

Plasma levels will usually decrease to an acceptable level within 48 hours after discontinuation of the medication; however, in severe cases involving acute renal failure, dialysis may be necessary.

Cognitive-Behavioral Therapy

Cognitive-behavioral therapy (CBT) focuses on the impact that thoughts have on behavior and feelings and encourages the child to use the power of rational thought to alter perceptions and behavior. This approach to counselling is usually short-term, about 12-20 sessions, with the first sessions to obtain a history, middle sessions to focus on problems, and last sessions to review and reinforce. Children are assigned "homework" during the sessions to practice new ways of thinking and to develop new coping strategies. The therapist helps the individual identify goals and then find ways to achieve those goals. CBT acknowledges that all problems cannot be resolved, but one can deal differently with problems. The therapist asks many questions to determine the child's areas of concern and encourages the child to question his/her own motivations and needs. CBT is goal-centered so each counselling session is structured toward a particular goal, such as coping techniques. CBT centers on the concept of unlearning previous behaviors and learning new ones, questioning behaviors, and doing homework.

Suicide

Suicide is the third leading cause of death among adolescents with about 1 million attempting suicide in the US each year. Additionally, antidepressants and atypical antipsychotics may increase suicidal ideation and depression.

Suicidal indications	High risk for repeated suicide attempt
• Depression or dysphoria. • Hostility to others. • Problems with peer relationships, and lack of close friends. • Post-crisis stress (divorce, death in family, graduation, college). • Withdrawn personality, • Quiet, lonely appearance, behavior. • Change in behavior (drop in grades, wearing black clothes, unkempt appearance, sleeping excessively, or not sleeping). • Co-morbid psychiatric problems (bipolar, schizophrenia). • Drug abuse.	Children who actually attempt suicide should be hospitalized and assessed for repeated suicide risk after initial treatment: • Violent suicide attempt (knives, gunshots). • Suicide attempt with low chance of rescue. • Ongoing psychosis or disordered thinking. • Ongoing severe depression and feeling of helplessness. • History of previous suicide attempts. • Lack of social support system.

Professional Caring and Ethical Practice

The ACCN Synergy Model

<u>Overview</u>
The ACCN Synergy model of nursing practice, developed by the ACCN for nursing certification, places the needs of the patient as a central focus and defines the relationship between 8 patient characteristics and 8 nurse competencies. These competencies and characteristics are evaluated on a scale (1-5).

Patient characteristics include resiliency, vulnerability, stability, complexity, resource availability, participation in care, participation in decision-making, and predictability.

Nurse competencies include clinical judgment, advocacy, caring practices, collaboration, systems thinking, response to diversity, clinical inquiry, and facilitation of learning.

The system or healthcare environment is the third element of the model. It provides support for the needs of the patients and empowers and nurtures the practice of nursing, caring, and ethical practice. All three of these systems are essential for Synergy. The needs of the patient are the driving force for nurse competencies and both are dependent on the healthcare system. When the needs, competencies, and system complement each other, Synergy is achieved, and outcomes for the nurse, the patient, and the system are optimized.

<u>Three Levels of Outcomes</u>
The ACCN Synergy model is based on three levels of quality outcomes (patient, nurse, and system). Six general indicators of quality outcomes include:
- Satisfaction of patient and family.
- Adverse incidents rates.
- Rate of complications.
- Adherence to discharge plans.
- Mortality rate.
- Length of stay in hospital.

These general outcomes are based on outcomes derived from the patient, the nurse, and the system:
- Patient outcomes include functional change, behavioral change, trust, ratings, satisfaction, comfort, and quality of life.
- Nurse outcomes include physiological changes, presence or absence of complications, extent to which care of treatment objectives were attained.
- System outcomes include recidivism, costs, and resource utilization.

Advocacy and Moral Agency

The ACCN Synergy Model

Nurse competencies under the ACCN Synergy model include advocacy/moral agency:

- Advocacy is working for the best interests of the patient despite personal values in conflict and assisting patients to have access to appropriate resources.
- Agency is openness and recognition of issues and a willingness to act.
- Moral agency is the ability to recognize needs and take action to influence the outcome of a conflict or decision.

The levels of advocacy/moral agency include:
- Level 1: This nurse works on behalf of the patient, assesses personal values, has awareness of patient's rights and ethical conflicts, and advocates for the patient when consistent with the nurse's personal values.
- Level 2: This nurse advocates for the patient/family, incorporates their values into the care plan even when they differ from the nurse's, and can utilize internal resources to assist patient/family with complex decisions.
- Level 3: This nurse advocates for patient/family despite differences in values and is able to utilize both internal and external resources to help to empower patient/family to make decisions.

Complementary Therapies

Complementary therapies, are used as well as conventional medical treatment and should be included if this is what the child/family wants, empowering them to take some control. Complementary therapies vary widely and most can easily be incorporated into the plan of care   The National Center for Complementary and Alternative Medicine recognizes the following:
- Whole medical systems include medical systems, such as homeopathic, naturopathic medicine, acupuncture, and Chinese herbal medications.
- Mind-body medicine can include support groups, medication, music, art, or dance therapy.
- Biologically-based practices include the use of food, vitamins, or nutrition for healing.
- Manipulative/body-based programs include massage or other types of manipulation, such as chiropractic treatment.

Energy therapies may be biofield therapies intended to affect the aura (energy field) that some believe surrounds all living things. These therapies include therapeutic touch and Reiki. Bioelectromagnetic-based therapies use a variety of magnetic fields.

Ethical Assessments

While the terms *ethics* and *morals* are sometimes used interchangeably, ethics is a study of morals and encompasses concepts of right and wrong. When making ethical assessments, one must consider not only what people should do but also what they actually do, as these two things are sometimes at odds. Ethical issues can be difficult to assess because of personal bias, and that is one of the reasons that sharing concerns with other internal sources and reaching consensus is so valuable. Issues of concern might include options for care, refusal of care, rights to privacy, adequate relief of suffering, and the right to self-determination.   Internal sources might include the ethics committee, whose charge is to make decisions regarding ethical issues. Risk management can provide guidance related to personal and institutional liability. External agencies might include government agencies, such as the public health department.

Beneficence and Nonmaleficence

Beneficence is an ethical principle that involves performing actions that are for the purpose of benefitting another person. In the care of a patient, any procedure or treatment should be done with the ultimate goal of benefitting the patient, and any actions that are not beneficial should be reconsidered. As a child ages and/or condition changes, procedures need to be continually reevaluated to determine if they are still of benefit.

Nonmaleficence is an ethical principle that means healthcare workers should provide care in a manner that does not cause direct intentional harm to the patient:
- The actual act must be good or morally neutral.
- The intent must be only for a good effect.
- A bad effect cannot serve as the means to get to a good effect.
- A good effect must have more benefit than a bad effect has harm.

Autonomy and Justice

Autonomy is the ethical principle that the individual has the right to make decisions about his/her own care. In the case of children or patients with dementia who cannot make autonomous decisions, parents or family members may serve as the legal decision maker. The nurse must keep the patient and/or family fully informed so that they can exercise their autonomy in informed decision-making.

Justice is the ethical principle that relates to the distribution of the limited resources of healthcare benefits to the members of society. These resources must be distributed fairly. This issue may arise if there is only one bed left and two sick patients. Justice comes into play in deciding which patient should stay and which should be transported or otherwise cared for. The decision should be made according to what is best or most just for the patients and not colored by personal bias.

Bioethics

Bioethics is a branch of ethics that involves making sure that the medical treatment given is the most morally correct choice given the different options that might be available and the differences inherent in the varied levels of treatment. In the acute/critical care unit, if the patients, parents, and the staff are in agreement when it comes to values and decision-making, then no ethical dilemma exists; however, when there is a difference in value beliefs between the patients/parents and the staff, there is a bioethical dilemma that must be resolved. Sometimes, discussion and explanation can resolve differences, but at times the institution's ethics committee must be brought in to resolve the conflict. The primary goal of bioethics is to determine the most morally correct action using the set of circumstances given.

Ensuring Patient/Family Rights

In order for patient/family rights to be incorporated into the plan of care, the care plan needs to be designed as a collaborative effort that encourages participation of patients and family members. There are a number of different programs that can be useful, such as including patients and families on advisory committees. Additionally, assessment tools, such as surveys for patients/families, can be utilized to gain insight in the issues that are important to them. While infants and small children cannot speak for themselves, "patient" is generally understood to include not only the immediate family but also other groups or communities who have an interest in the care of an individual or individuals. Because many hospital stays are now short-term, programs that include follow-up interviews and assessments are especially valuable in determining if the needs of the patient/family were addressed in the care plan.

Confidentiality

Confidentiality is the obligation that is present in a professional-patient relationship. Nurses are under an obligation to protect the information they possess concerning the family whose child they are caring for. Care should be taken in the critical care unit to safeguard that information and provide the privacy that the family deserves. This is accomplished through the use of required passwords when parents call for information about their children and through the limitation of who is allowed to visit a child (usually restricted to only those who accompany parents). There may be times when confidentiality must be broken to save the life of a patient, but those circumstances are rare. The critical care nurse must make all efforts to safeguard patient records and identification. Computerized record keeping should be done in such a way that the screen is not visible to others, and paper records must be secured.

<u>Issues Related to a Child's Desire for Confidentiality</u>
Children, especially adolescents, may have confidentiality concerns in relation to their health or activities that they do not want divulged to their parents. Young people may be uncomfortable addressing concerns verbally and may be more forthcoming if given a questionnaire to fill out as a beginning point for discussion. The critical care nurse is often faced with ethical concerns about dealing with confidentiality, but the best course is to deal with the issue directly by informing children that what they say will be held in confidence within certain limitations:

- Mandatory reporting requirements must be upheld, including reports of child abuse, sexual abuse, and communicable diseases.
- Health endangerment, such as through the abuse of drugs or alcohol, eating disorders, or suicidal thoughts, must be reported to the parents, while assuring the child that the critical care nurse will be there to support and help them to discuss these matters with parents.

Informed Consent

Parents/guardians of children must provide informed consent for all treatment the child receives. This includes a thorough explanation of all procedures and treatment and associated risks. Parents/guardians should be apprised of all options and allowed input on the type of treatments. Parents/guardians should be apprised of all reasonable risks and any complications that might be life threatening or increase morbidity. The American Medical Association has established guidelines for informed consent:

- Explanation of diagnosis.
- Nature and reason for treatment or procedure.
- Risks and benefits.
- Alternative options (regardless of cost or insurance coverage).
- Risks and benefits of alternative options.
- Risks and benefits of not having a treatment or procedure.
- Providing informed consent is a requirement of all states.

Self Advocacy of Patients / Families

Empowering patients and families to act as their own advocates requires they have a clear understanding of their rights and responsibilities. These should be given (in print form) and/or presented (audio/video) to patients and families on admission or as soon as possible:

- Rights should include competent, non-discriminatory medical care that respects privacy and allows participation in decisions about care and the right to refuse care. They should have clear understandable explanations of treatments, options, and conditions, including outcomes. They should be apprised of transfers, changes in care plan, and advance directives. They should have access to medical records information about charges.
- Responsibilities should including providing honest and thorough information about health issues and medical history. They should ask for clarification if they don't understand information that is provided to them, and they should follow the plan of care that is outlined or explain why that is not possible. They should treat staff and other patients with respect.

Advance Directives

In accordance to Federal and state laws, individuals have the right to self-determination in health care, including decisions about end of life care through advance directives such as living wills and the right to assign a surrogate person to make decisions through a durable power of attorney. Parents/guardians have the right to make these decisions for minors. Parents/guardians should routinely be questioned about an advanced directive as they may present at a healthcare organization without the document. If parents/guardians indicate the desire for a do-not-resuscitate (DNR) order for a seriously ill child, that child should not receive resuscitative treatments for terminal illness or conditions in which meaningful recovery cannot occur. For those with DNR requests or that withdrawing life support, staff should provide the child palliative rather than curative measures, such as pain control and/or oxygen, and emotional support to the child and family. Religious traditions and beliefs about death should be treated with respect.

Caring Practices

The ACCN Synergy Model

In the ACCN Synergy model, caring practices encompass all nursing activities that respond to the individual patient's and family's needs in a caring, compassionate, and therapeutic environment to promote patient comfort and prevent unnecessary suffering. Caring practices recognize inner strength and its relation to healing and seek to enhance the dignity of the individual through vigilance, nurturing, and skilled technical and basic nursing practices. Levels of caring practices include:

- Level 1: This nurse provides a safe environment and cares for the present basic needs of the patient without focus on future needs and considers death a potential outcome.
- Level 3: This nurse provides compassionate care, responding to changes in the patient and acts of kindness while accepting death as a possible outcome and providing measures to ensure good end-of-life care and a peaceful death.
- Level 5: This nurse is fully engaged in patient care and understands and interprets patient/family dynamics and needs, ensuring comfort, dignity, and safety while respecting the individual and family.

Problem-Solving Steps

- Problem solving to anticipate or prevent recurrences of patient/family dissatisfaction involves arriving at a hypothesis, testing, and assessing data to determine if the hypothesis holds true. If a problem has arisen, taking steps to resolve the immediate problem is only the first step if recurrence is to be avoided:The issue: Talk with the patient or family and staff to determine if the problem related to a failure of communication or other issues, such as culture or religion.
- Collect data: This may mean interviewing additional staff or reviewing documentation, gaining a variety of perspectives.Important concepts: Determine if there are issues related to values or beliefs.
- Consider reasons for actions: Distinguish between motivation and intention on the part of all parties to determine the reason for the problem.
- Make a decision: A decision on how to prevent a recurrence of a problem should be based on advocacy and moral agency, reaching the best solution possible for the patient and family.

Patients'/Families' Rights

Patients' (families') rights in relation to what they should expect from a healthcare organization are outlined in both standards of the Joint Commission and National Committee for Quality Assurance.

Rights include:
- Respect for patient, including personal dignity and psychosocial, spiritual, and cultural considerations.
- Response to needs related to access and pain control.
- Ability to make decisions about care, including informed consent, advance directives, and end of life care.

- Procedure for registering complaints or grievances.
- Protection of confidentiality and privacy.
- Freedom from abuse or neglect.
- Protection during research and information related to ethical issues of research.
- Appraisal of outcomes, including unexpected outcomes.
- Information about organization, services, and practitioners.
- Appeal procedures for decisions regarding benefits and quality of care.
- Organizational code of ethical behavior.
- Procedures for donating and procuring organs/tissue.

Facilitating Safe Passage

Facilitating safe passage is part of caring practice that ensures patient safety, in a broad sense, from a variety of perspectives:
- Giving appropriate medications and treatment without errors that endanger the child's health is essential.
- Providing information to the patient/family about treatments, changes, conditions, and other aspects related to care helps them to cope with the situations as they arise.
- Preventing infection is central to patient safety and includes staff using proper infection control methods, such as handwashing.
- Knowing the person requires the nurse to take the time and effort to understand the needs and wishes of the patient/family.
- Assisting with transitions involves not only helping the patient/family cope with moving from one form of treatment, or one unit to another but also with transitions in health, such as from illness to health or from illness to death.

End-Of-Life Palliative Care

The World Health Organization (WHO) defines end-of-life and palliative care as active total care of patient whose disease is no longer responsive to treatment. Palliative care, especially pain management, is often delayed or inadequate in pediatric patients. The dying child and parents/family must be considered a unit when planning for care, and a multidisciplinary approach that includes physicians, nurses, social workers, and chaplains or spiritual guides can help the family through this difficult period. Parents/family may equate pain medication with euthanasia or assisted suicide. Additionally, parents/family may feel that the child's increased sedation robs them of time with the child or may fear addiction. These concerns must be respected, but providing adequate information and support while allowing the parents/family to express their feelings can often allay many of these fears.

Parents/Family of Dying Child

Before Death
Parents/families of dying children often do not receive adequate support from nursing staff who feel unprepared for dealing with parents'/families' grief and unsure of how provide comfort, but parents/families are in desperate need of this support:

Before death	• Stay with the family and sit quietly, allowing them to talk, cry, or interact if they desire.
	• Avoid platitudes: "His suffering will be over soon."
	• Avoid judgmental reactions to what family members say or do and realize that anger, fear, guilt, and irrational behavior are normal responses to acute grief and stress.
	• Show caring by touching the child and encouraging family to do the same.
	• Note: Touching hands, arms, or shoulders of family members can provide comfort, but follow clues of the family.
	• Provide referrals to support groups if available.

At Death and After
Parents/families of dying children require much support:

Time of death	Reassure family that all measures have been taken to ensure the child's comfort.
	Express personal feeling of loss, "She was such a sweet child, and I'll miss her" and allow family to express feelings and memories.
	Provide information about what is happening during the dying process, explaining death rales, Cheyne-Stokes respirations, etc.
	Alert family members to imminent death if they are not present. Assist to contact clergy/spiritual advisors.
	Respect feelings and needs of parents, siblings, and other family.
After death	Encourage parents/family members to stay with the child as long as they wish to hold the child and/or say goodbye. Use the child's name when talking to the family. Assist them to make arrangements, such as contacting funeral home. If an autopsy is required, discuss with the family and explain when it will take place. If organ donation is to occur, assist the family to make arrangements. Encourage family members to grieve and express emotions.
	Send card or condolence note.

Kübler-Ross's Five Stages of Grief

Denial and Anger
Grief is a normal response to the death or severe illness/abnormality of an infant or child. How a person deals with grief is very personal, and each person will grieve differently. Elisabeth Kübler-Ross identified five stages of grief in *On Death and Dying* (1969). A person may not go through each stage but usually goes through two of the five stages:

• Denial: The parents may be resistive to information and unable to accept that a child is dying/impaired or believe that the child is not theirs. They may act stunned, immobile, or detached and may be unable to respond appropriately or remember what's said, often repeatedly asking the same questions.

- Anger: As reality becomes clear, parents may react with pronounced anger, directed inward or outward. Women, especially, may blame themselves and self-anger may lead to severe depression and guilt, assuming they are to blame because of some action before or during pregnancy. Outward anger, more common in men, may be expressed as overt hostility.

<u>Bargaining, Depression, and Acceptance</u>
Kübler-Ross's five stages of grief (in addition to denial and anger):
- Bargaining: This involves if-then thinking (often directed at a deity): "If I go to church every way, then God will prevent this." Parents may change doctors, trying to change the outcome.
- Depression: As the parents begin to accept the loss, they may become depressed, feeling no one understands and overwhelmed with sadness. They may be tearful or crying and may withdraw or ask to be left alone.
- Acceptance: This final stage represents a form of resolution and often occurs outside of the medical environment after months. Parents are able to resume their normal activities and lose the constant preoccupation with their child. They are able to think of the child without severe pain. With a disabled child, acceptance may be delayed because of daily challenges and reminders.

Types of Grief

Anticipatory grief occurs when a child is diagnosed with a terminal illness. The parent begins to mourn over the loss of the child before he or she expires.

Incongruent grief occurs when the mother and the father are "out of synch" in their grieving process, stressing their relationship. It may be due to the differences in how men and women grieve, or it may be because the woman typically bonds with the infant during the pregnancy, while the father bonds after the child is born, and this bonding may take place less readily if an infant remains hospitalized after birth.

Delayed grief occurs when the grieving process is postponed months to years after the loss of a child. Initially, the parent may not be able to grieve appropriately, because of an inability to cope or the pressing need to care for other family members.

Safety Related to Medication Errors

There are about 7000 deaths yearly in the United States attributed to medication errors. Studies indicate that there are errors in 1 in 5 doses of medication given to patients in hospitals. A caring environment is one in which patient safety is ensured with proper handling and administering of medications:
- Avoiding error-prone abbreviations or symbols. The Joint Commission has established a list of abbreviations to avoid, but mistakes are frequent with other abbreviations as well. In many cases, abbreviations and symbols should be avoided altogether or restricted to a limited approved list.
- Preventing errors from illegible handwriting. Handwritten orders should be block printed to reduce change of error.
- Instituting bar coding and scanners that allow the patient's wristband and medications to be scanned for verification.

- Providing lists of similarly-named medications to educate staff.
- Establishing an institutional policy for administering of medications that includes protocols for verification of drug, dosage, and patient as well as educating the patient about the medications.

Pediatric Safety Measures During Hospitalization

Environment and Toys

Pediatric safety measures during hospitalization	
Room & equipment	• Windows must be secured and cords out of reach. • Electrical outlets are covered and electrical equipment secured and out of arms' reach. • Small items, which may choke a child, must be disposed of properly. • Furniture (such as bed size) should be appropriate for age/size of child. • Crib sides must be up and secured and if caring for a child with the side rail down, the nurse should never turn away and should always keep a hand on the child. • Infants/toddlers who can climb should have a crib with a protective dome. • Beds of older children should be locked so they don't slide.
Toys	• Toys should be clean, non-allergenic, washable, and unbreakable. • Balloons and toys with small parts should be avoided with small children. • If oxygen is in use, electrical or friction toys should be avoided.

Surveillance and Transportation

Pediatric safety measures during hospitalization	
Surveillance	• The nurse must always know where children are, and ambulatory children must be clear about where they can go and cannot go. These limitations must be strictly enforced because access to elevators, laundry chutes, or restricted work areas could pose risks for the child or others. • The child should be provided with supervised activities to reduce boredom. • Parents should be asked to notify staff when they arrive at and leave the unit.

Transportation	• Infants and very small children may be carried for short distances within the unit itself with football, horizontal-thigh grasp, or vertical back support hold, but for longer distances, the child should be transported in a safe and appropriate manner, such as in a basinet or crib.
	• Older children are transported in wheelchairs (with safety belt if necessary) or gurneys with side rails.

Therapeutic Communication

Introduction, Encouragement, and Empathy
Therapeutic communication begins with respect for the patient/family and the assumption that all communication, verbal and non-verbal, has meaning. Listening must be done empathetically.

Techniques that facilitate communication include:

Intro-duction	Make a personal introduction and use the patient's name: "Joey, I am Susan Williams, your nurse."
Encour-agement	Use an open-ended opening statement: "Is there anything you'd like to discuss?"
	Acknowledge comments: "Yes," and "I understand."
	Allow silence and observe non-verbal behavior rather than trying to force conversation.
	Ask for clarification if statements are unclear.
	Refect statements back (use sparingly):
	• Patient: "I hate this hospital."
	• Nurse: "You hate this hospital?"
Empathy	Make observations: "You are shaking," and "You seem worried."
	Recognize feelings:
	• Patient: "I want to go home."
	• Nurse: "It must be hard to be away from your home and family."
	Provide information as honestly and completely as possible about condition, treatment, and procedures and respond to patient's questions and concerns.

Exploration, Orientation, Collaboration, and Validation
Methods to promote a caring and supportive environment with therapeutic communication include:

Exploration	Verbally express implied messages:
	• Patient: "This treatment is a waste of time."
	• Nurse: "You think the treatment isn't helping you?"
	Explore a topic but allow the patient to terminate the discussion without further probing: "I'd like to hear how you feel about that.

Orientation	Indicate reality: • Patient: "Someone is screaming." • Nurse: "That sound was an ambulance siren." Comment on distortions without directly agreeing or disagreeing: • Patient: "That nurse promised I didn't have to walk again." • Nurse: "Really? That's surprising because the doctor ordered physical therapy twice a day."
Collaboration	Work together to achieve better results: "Maybe if we talk about this, we can figure out a way to make the treatment easier for you."
Validation	Seek validation: "Do you feel better now?" or "Did the medication help you breathe better."

Avoiding Non-Therapeutic Communication

<u>Using Language Ineffectively, Providing Inappropriate Advice/Approval, and Asking or Agreeing Inappropriately</u>
While using therapeutic communication is important, it is equally important to avoid interjecting non-therapeutic communication, which can effectively block effective communication.

Avoid the following:
- Meaningless clichés: "Don't worry. Everything will be fine." "Isn't it a nice day?"
- Providing advice: "You should…" or "The best thing to do is…." It's better when patients ask for advice to provide facts and encourage the patient to reach a decision.
- Inappropriate approval that prevents the patient from expressing true feeling or concerns:
  - Patient: "I shouldn't cry."
  - Nurse: "That's right! You're a big girl!"
- Asking for explanations of behavior that is not directly related to patient care and requires analysis and explanation of feelings: "Why are you upset?"
- Agreeing with rather than accepting and responding to patient's statements can make it difficult for the patient to change his/her statement or opinion later: "I agree with you," or "You are right."

<u>Negative and Inappropriate Responses</u>
Methods to promote a caring and supportive environment, avoiding non-therapeutic communication include:
- Negative judgments: "You should stop arguing with the nurses."
- Devaluing patient's feelings: "Everyone gets upset at times."
- Disagreeing directly: "That can't be true," or "I think you are wrong."
- Defending against criticism: "The doctor is not being rude; he's just very busy tody."
- Subject change to avoid dealing with uncomfortable topics;
  - Patient: "I'm never going to get well."
  - Nurse: "Your family will be here in just a few minutes."
- Inappropriate literal responses, even as a joke, especially if the patient is at all confused or having difficulty expressing ideas:

- Patient: "There are bugs crawling under my skin."
- Nurse: "I'll get some buy spray,"
- Challenge to establish reality often just increases confusion and frustration:
  - "If you were dying, you wouldn't be able to yell and kick!"

Collaboration

The ACCN Synergy Model

In the ACCN Synergy model, collaboration is a team approach of working with a variety of others (physicians, nurses, dieticians, therapist, families, social workers, community leaders and members, clergy, intra- and inter-disciplinary teams) in a cooperative manner, using good therapeutic communication skills, to ensure that each person is contributing optimally toward reaching patient goals and positive outcomes. Collaboration requires mutual respect, professional maturity, common purpose, and a positive sense of self.

Levels of collaboration include:
- Level 1: This nurse participates in collaborative activities, learns from others, including mentors, and respects the input of others.
- Level 3: This nurse not only participates in collaborative activities but also initiates them and actively seeks learning opportunities.
- Level 5: This nurse takes a leadership role in collaborative activities by mentoring and teaching others while still seeking learning opportunities and actively seeks additional resources as needed.

Skills Needed for Collaboration

Nurses must learn the set of skills needed for collaboration in order to move nursing forward. Nurses must take an active role in gathering data for evidence-based practice to support nursing's role in health care and must share this information with other nurses and health professionals in order to plan staffing levels and to provide optimal care to patients. Increased and adequate staffing has consistently been shown to reduce adverse outcomes, but there is a well-documented shortage of nurses in the United States, and more than half of current RNs work outside the hospital. Increased patient loads not only increase adverse outcomes but also increase job dissatisfaction and burnout. In order to manage the challenges facing nursing, nurses must develop skills needed for collaboration:
- Be willing to compromise.
- Communicate clearly. Specific challenges and problems.
- Focus on the task.
- Work with teams.

Delegation of Tasks

The scope of nursing practice includes delegation of tasks to unlicensed assistive personnel, providing those personnel have adequate training and knowledge to carry out the tasks. Delegation should be used to manage the workload and to provide adequate and safe care. The nurse who delegates remains accountable for patient outcomes and for supervision of the person to whom the task was delegated, so the nurse must consider the following:

- Whether knowledge, skills, and training of the unlicensed assistive personnel provides the ability to perform the delegated task.
- Whether the patient's condition and needs have been properly evaluated and assessed.
- Whether the nurse is able to provide ongoing supervision.

Delegation should be done in a manner that reduces liability by providing adequate communication. This includes specific directions about the task, including what needs to be done, when, and for how long. Expectations related to consultation, reporting, and completion of tasks should be clearly defined. The nurse should be available to assist if necessary.

Discuss 5 Rights of Delegation

Prior to delegating tasks, the nurse should assess the needs of the patients and determine the task that needs to be completed, assure that he/she can remain accountable and can supervise the task appropriately and evaluate effective completion.

The 5 rights of delegation include:
- Right task: The nurse should determine an appropriate task to delegate for a specific patient.
- Right circumstance: The nurse has considered the setting, resources, time factors, safety factors, and all other relevant information to determine the appropriateness of delegation.
- Right person: The nurse is in the right position to choose the right person (by virtue of education/skills) to perform a task for the right patient.
- Right direction: The nurse provides a clear description of the task, the purpose, any limits, and expected outcomes.
- Right supervision: The nurse is able to supervise, intervene as needed, and evaluate performance of the task.

Delegation Of Tasks In Teams

On major responsibility of leadership and management in performance improvement teams is using delegation effectively. The purpose of having a team is so that the work is shared, and leaders can cripple themselves by taking on too much of the workload. Additionally, failure to delegate shows an inherent distrust in team members.

Delegation includes:
- Assessing the skills and available time of the team members, determining if a task is suitable for an individual.
- Assigning tasks, with clear instructions that include explanation of objectives and expectations, including a timeline.
- Ensuring that the tasks are completed properly and on time by monitoring progress but not micromanaging.
- Reviewing the final results and recording outcomes.

Because the leader is ultimately responsible for the delegated work, mentoring, monitoring, and providing feedback and intervention as necessary during this process is a necessary component of leadership. While delegated tasks may not always be completed successfully, they represent an opportunity for learning.

Creating a Common Vision of Care

Facilitating the creation of a common vision for care within the healthcare system begins with the organization/facility, working collaboratively to create teams and an organization focused on serving the patient/family. A common vision should be the ideal in any organization, but achieving such a goal requires a true collaborative effort:

- Inclusion of all levels of staff across the organization/facility, both those in nursing and non-nursing positions.
- Consensus building through discussions, inservice, and team meetings to bring about convergence of diverse viewpoints.
- Facilitation that values creativity and provides encouragement during the process.
- Vision statement incorporating the common vision that accessible to all staff.

Recognition that a common vision is an organic concept that may evolve over time and should be reevaluated regularly and changed as needed to reflect the needs of the organization, patients, families, and staff.

Teambuilding

Leading, facilitating, and participating in performance improvement teams requires a thorough understanding of the dynamics of team building:

- Initial interactions: This is the time when members begin to define their roles and develop relationships, determining if they are comfortable in the group.
- Power issues: The members observe the leader and determine who controls the meeting and how control is exercised, beginning to form alliances.
- Organizing: Methods to achieve work are clarified and team members begin to work together, gaining respect for each other's contributions and working toward a common goal.
- Team identification: Interactions often become less formal as members develop rapport, and members are more willing to help and support each other to achieve goals.
- Excellence: This develops through a combination of good leadership, committed team members, clear goals, high standards, external recognition, spirit of collaboration, and a shared commitment to the process.

Techniques for Effective Team Meetings

Leading and facilitating improvement teams requires utilizing good techniques for meetings. Considerations include:

- Scheduling: Both the time and the place must be convenient and conducive to working together, so the leader must review the work schedules of those involved, finding the most convenient time. Venues or meeting rooms should allow for sitting in a circle or around a table to facilitate equal exchange of ideas. Any necessary technology, such as computers or overhead projectors, or other equipment, such as whiteboards, should be available.

- Preparation: The leader should prepare a detailed agenda that includes a list of items for discussion.
- Conduction: Each item of the agenda should be discussed, soliciting input from all group members. Tasks should be assigned to individual members based on their interest and part in the process in preparation for the next meeting. The leader should summarize input and begin a tentative future agenda.
- Observation: The leader should observe the interactions, including verbal and non-verbal communication, and respond to these.

Coordination of Intra-and Inter-Disciplinary Teams

There are a number of skills that are needed to lead and facilitate coordination of intra- and inter-disciplinary teams:
- Communicating openly is essential with all members encouraged to participate as valued members of a cooperative team.
- Avoiding interrupting or interpreting the point another is trying to make allows free flow of ideas.
- Avoiding jumping to conclusions, which can effectively shut off communication.
- Active listening requires paying attentions and asking questions for clarification rather than to challenge other's ideas.
- Respecting others opinions and ideas, even when opposed to one's own, is absolutely essential.
- Reacting and responding to facts rather than feelings allows one to avoid angry confrontations or diffuse anger.
- Clarifying information or opinions stated can help avoid misunderstandings.
- Keeping unsolicited advice out of the conversation shows respect for others and allows them to solicit advice without feeling pressured.

Leadership Styles

Charismatic, Bureaucratic, Autocratic, and Consultative
Leadership styles often influence the perception of leadership values and commitment to collaboration. There are a number of different leadership styles:

Charismatic	Depends upon personal charisma to influence people, and may be very persuasive, but this type leader may engage "followers" and relate to one group rather than the organization at large, limiting effectiveness.
Bureaucratic	Follows organization rules exactly and expects everyone else to do so. This is most effective in handling cash flow or managing work in dangerous work environments. This type of leadership may engender respect but may not be conducive to change.
Autocratic	Makes decisions independently and strictly enforces rules, but team members often feel left out of process and may not be supportive. This type of leadership is most effective in crisis situations, but may have difficulty gaining commitment of staff
Consultative	Presents a decision and welcomes input and questions although decisions rarely change. This type of leadership is most effective when gaining the support of staff is critical to the success of

	proposed changes.

Participatory, Democratic, and Laissez-Faire
Different leadership styles in developing leadership values and commitment to collaboration include:

Participatory	Presents a potential decision and then makes final decision based on input from staff or teams. This type of leadership is time-consuming and may result in compromises that are not wholly satisfactory to management or staff, but this process is motivating to staff who feel their expertise is valued.
Democratic	Presents a problem and asks staff or teams to arrive at a solution although the leader usually makes the final decision. This type of leadership may delay decision-making, but staff and teams are often more committed to the solutions because of their input.
Laissez-faire (free rein)	Exerts little direct control but allows employees/ teams to make decisions with little interference. This may be effective leadership if teams are highly skilled and motivated, but in many cases this type of leadership is the product of poor management skills and little is accomplished because of this lack of leadership.

Resistance To Organizational Change

Performance improvement processes cannot occur without organizational change, and resistance to change is common for many people, so coordinating collaborative processes requires anticipating resistance and taking steps to achieve cooperation. Resistance often relates to concerns about job loss, increased responsibilities, and general denial or lack of understanding and frustration. Leaders can prepare others involved in the process of change by taking these steps:

- Be honest, informative, and tactful, giving people thorough information about anticipated changes and how the changes will affect them, including positives.
- Be patient in allowing people the time they need to contemplate changes and express anger or disagreement.
- Be empathetic in listening carefully to the concerns of others.
- Encourage participation, allowing staff to propose methods of implementing change, so they feel some sense of ownership.
- Establish a climate in which all staff members are encouraged to identify the need for change on an ongoing basis.
- Present further ideas for change to management.

Conflict Resolution

Conflict is an almost inevitable product of teamwork, and the leader must assume responsibility for conflict resolution. While conflicts can be disruptive, they can produce positive outcomes by forcing team members to listen to different perspectives and opening dialogue. The team should make a plan for dealing with conflict resolution. The best time for conflict resolution is when differences emerge but before open conflict and hardening of positions occur. The leader must pay close attention to the people and problems involved, listen carefully, and reassure those involved that their points of view are understood. Steps to conflict resolution include:

- Allow both sides to present their side of conflict without bias, maintaining a focus on opinions rather than individuals.
- Encourage cooperation through negotiation and compromise.
- Maintain the focus, providing guidance to keep the discussions on track and avoid arguments.
- Evaluate the need for renegotiation, formal resolution process, or third party.
- Utilize humor and empathy to diffuse escalating tensions.
- Summarize the issues, outlining key arguments.
- Avoid forcing resolution if possible

Collaboration Between Nurse and Patient/Family

One of the most important forms of collaboration is that between the nurse and the patient/family, but this type of collaboration is often overlooked. Nurses and others in the healthcare team must always remember that the point of collaborating is to improve patient care, and this means that the patient and patient's family must remain central to all planning. For example, including family in planning for a patient takes time initially, but sitting down and asking the patient and family, "What do you want?" and using the Synergy model to evaluate patient's (and family's) characteristics can provide valuable information that saves time in the long run and facilitates planning and expenditure of resources. Families, and even young children, often want to participate in care and planning and feel validated and more positive toward the medical system when they are included.

Communication Skills for Collaboration

Collaboration requires a number of communication skills that differ from those involved in communication between nurse and patient. These skills include:

- Using an assertive approach: It's important for the nurse to honestly express opinions and to state them clearly and with confidence, but the nurse must do so in a calm non-threatening manner.
- Making casual conversation: It's easier to communicate with people with whom one has a personal connection. Asking open-ended questions, asking about other's work, or commenting on someone's contributions helps to establish a relationship. The time before meetings, during breaks, and after meetings presents an opportunity for this type of conversation.
- Being competent in public speaking: Collaboration requires that a nurse be comfortable speaking and presenting ideas to groups of people, and doing so helps the person to gain credibility. This is a skill that must be practiced.
- Communicating in writing: The written word remains a critical component of communication, and the nurse should be able to communicate clearly and grammatically.

Systems Thinking

The ACCN Synergy Model

In the ACCN Synergy model, systems thinking is having the background knowledge and practical tools to manage both environmental and system resources, within and outside of the healthcare system, in order to solve problems for the patient/family and meet their needs. Solving problems requires a holistic view of the interrelationships and understanding of how structures, patterns, and events affect outcomes. Levels of systems thinking include:

- Level 1: This nurse views himself/herself as the primary resource to meet the needs of the patient within the confines of the unit and doesn't recognize the need to negotiate.
- Level 3: This nurse looks beyond the unit and personal contributions to care to view the patient's progress through the entire system and sees the need to negotiate with others to provide the best resources available although may lack the skills needed to do so,
- Level 5: This nurse is expert at understanding the organization holistically and uses a number of different strategies to negotiate with others and assist the patient with progress through the system.

Patient Characteristics
The ACCN Synergy method for patient care recognizes that there are a number of patient characteristics that must be considered if a nurse's competencies are to match those of the patient/family:

- Resiliency is the ability to recover from a devastating illness and regain a sense of stability, both physically and emotionally. Things that often support resiliency are faith, a positive sense of hope, and a supportive network of friends and family.
- Vulnerability are those factors putting a person at increased risk and interfering with recovery and/or compliance, such as anxiety, fear, lack of support, chronic illness, prejudice, and lack of information.
- Stability allows a patient/family to maintain a state of equilibrium (physically and/or emotionally) despite illness and challenges. Important factors include relief from stress, conflicts, or emotional burdens, motivation, and values.
- Complexity occurs when more than one system is involved, and these can be internal (cardiac and renal systems) or external (addicted and homeless) or some combination (ill with poor family dynamics).

Barriers to System Thinking

Identification With Role, Victimization, and Relying on Past Experience
Barriers to system thinking can arise with the individual, the department, or the administrative level:

- Identification with role rather than purpose: People see themselves from the perspective of their role in the system, as nurse or physician, and are not able to step outside their preconceived ideas to view situations holistically or to accept the roles of others. They may lack the ability to look at situations as human beings first, and professionals second.

- Feelings of victimization: People may blame the organization or the leadership for personal shortcomings or feel that there is nothing that they can do to improve or change situations. A feeling of victimization may permeate an institution to the point that meaningful communication cannot take place, and people are not open to change.
- Relying on past experience: New directions require new solutions, so being mired in the past or relying solely on past experience can prevent progress.

Autocratic Views, Failure to Adapt, and Weak Consensus

Barriers to system thinking include:
- Autocratic views: Some feel that their perceptions and practices are the only ones that are acceptable and often have a narrow focus so that they cannot view the system as a whole but focus on short-term outcomes. They fail to see that there are many aspects to a problem, affecting many parts of the system.
- Failure to adapt: Change is difficult for many individuals and institutions, but the medical world is changing rapidly, and this requires adaptability. Those who fail to adapt may feel threatened by changes and unsure of their ability to relearn new concepts, principles, and procedures.
- Weak consensus: Groups that arrive at easy or weak consensus without delving into important issues may delude themselves into believing that they have solved problems and remain fixed and often ignored rather than moving forward.

Delivery of Care

Impact of Social, Political, Regulatory, and Economic Forces on The Delivery of Care.

The delivery of care is impacted by a numerous forces:
- Social forces are increasing demand for access to treatment and medical services, both traditional and complementary. As society views equitable medical care as a right, then delivery of care must be available to all.
- Political forces affect medical care as the Federal and state governments increasingly become purchasers of medical care, imposing their guidelines and limitations on the medical system.
- Regulatory forces may be local, state, or Federal and can have a profound effect of delivery of care and services, differing from one state or region to another.
- Economic forces, such as managed care or cost-containment committees, try to contain costs to insurers and facilities by controlling access to and duration of treatment, and limiting products. Economic pressure is working to prevent duplication of services in a geographical area, and providers are creating networks to purchase supplies and equipment directly.

Concepts of Systems Thinking

The promotion of organizational values and commitment requires that the organization embody systems thinking and the associated concepts. Systems thinking focuses on how systems interrelate, with each part affecting the entire system.

Concepts include:
- Individual responsibility: Individuals are encouraged to establish their own goals within the organization and to work toward a purpose.

- Learning process: The internalized beliefs of the staff are respected while building upon these beliefs to establish a mindset based on continuous learning and improvement.
- Vision: A sharing of organizational vision helps staff to understand the purpose of change and builds commitment.
- Team process: Teams are assisted to develop good listening and collaborative skills so that there is an increase in dialogue and an ability to reach consensus.
- Systems thinking: Staff members are encouraged to understand the interrelationship of all members of the organization and to appreciate how any change affects the whole.

Steps to Systems Thinking

An approach to systems thinking is especially valuable in organizations in which there is lack of consensus, effective change is stalemated, and standards are inconsistent. Systems thinking is a critical thinking approach to problem solving that takes an organization-wide perspective.

Steps include:
- The issue: Describe the problem in detail without judgment or solutions.Behavior patterns: This includes listing factors related to the problem, using graphs to outline possible trends.
- Establish cause-effect relationships: This may include using the Five Whys or other root cause analysis or feedback loops.Patterns of performance/behavior: Determine how variables affect outcomes and the types of patterns of behavior currently taking place.
- Find solutions: Discuss possible solutions and outcomes.
- Institute performance improvement activities: Make changes and then monitor for changes in behavior.

Key Quality Concepts

There are a number of key concepts related to quality that must be communicated to all members of an organization through inservice, workshops, newsletters, fact sheets, and team meetings. Quality care/performance should be:
- Appropriate to needs and in keeping with best practices.
- Accessible to the individual despite financial, cultural, or other barriers.
- Competent, with practitioners well-trained and adhering to standards.
- Coordinated among all healthcare providers.
- Effective in achieving outcomes based on the current state of knowledge.
- Efficient in methods of achieving the desired outcomes.
- Preventive, allowing for early detection and prevention of problems.
- Respectful and caring with consideration of the individual needs given primary importance.
- Safe so that the organization is free of hazards or dangers that may put patients or others at risk.

Response to Diversity

The ACCN Synergy Model

In the ACCN Synergy model, response to diversity is the ability to recognize a wide range of differences (social, cultural, ethnic, racial, and economic, language, religious), to appreciate these differences and incorporate consideration for them into the plan of care. Diverse groups also include the disabled, gay and lesbians, and marginal groups, such as the homeless. Levels of response to diversity include:

- Level 1: This nurse can assess diversity with standardized questionnaires and provide care based on personal belief system and past experience, but doesn't seek assistance in dealing adequately with diversity.
- Level 3: This nurse takes a much more active role in asking about issues of diversity issues and incorporates needs into the plan of care, teaching the patient about the healthcare system.
- Level 5: This nurse considers issues of diversity in all aspects of care and presents patients with alternatives, responding to, anticipating, and integrating consideration of cultural and other differences.

Cultural Competence

Difference cultures view health and illness from very different perspectives, and patients often come from a mix of many cultures, so the acute care nurse must be not only accepting of cultural differences but must be sensitive and aware. There are a number of characteristics that are important for a nurse to have cultural competence:

- Appreciating diversity: This must be grounded in information about other cultures and understanding of their value system.
- Assessing own cultural perspectives: Self-awareness is essential to understanding potential biases.
- Understanding intercultural dynamics: This must include understanding ways in which cultures cooperate, differ, communicate, and reach understanding.
- Recognizing institutional culture: Each institutional unit (hospital, clinic, office) has an inherent set of values that may be unwritten but is accepted by the staff.
- Adapting patient service to diversity: This is the culmination of cultural competence as it s the point of contact between cultures.

Blood Products and Jehovah Witnesses

Jehovah Witnesses have traditionally shunned transfusions and blood products as part of their religious belief. In 2004, the *Watchtower,* a Jehovah Witness publication presented a guide for members. When medical care indicates the need for blood transfusion or blood products and the patient and/or family members are practicing Jehovah Witnesses, this may present a conflict. It's important to approach the patient/family with full information and reasons for the transfusion or blood components without being judgmental, allowing them to express their feelings. In fact, studies show that while adults often refuse transfusions for themselves, they frequently allow their children to receive blood products, so one should never assume that an individual would refuse blood products based on the religion alone. Jehovah Witnesses can receive fractionated blood cells, thus allowing hemoglobin-based blood substitutes. The following guidelines are provided to church members:

Basic blood standards for Jehovah Witnesses	
Not acceptable	Whole blood: red cells, white cells, platelets, plasma
Acceptable	Fractions from red cells, white cells, platelets, and plasma

Mexican Patients

Religion, Families, Language, and Emotions

Many areas of the country have large populations of Mexican and Mexican-Americans. As always, it's important to recognize that cultural generalizations don't always apply to individuals. Recent immigrants, especially, have cultural needs that the nurse must understand:

- Many Mexicans are Catholic and may like the nurse to make arrangements for a priest to visit.
- Large extended families may come to visit to support the patient and family, so patients should receive clear explanations about how many visitors are allowed, but some flexibility may be required.
- Language barriers may exist as some may have limited or no English skills so translation services should be available around the clock.
- Mexican culture encourages outward expressions of emotions, so family may react strongly to news about a patient's condition, and people who are ill may expect some degree of pampering, so extra attention to the patient/family members may alleviate some of their anxiety.

Education, Time Perception, Assertiveness, Folk Medicine, Children and Women

Caring for Mexican and Mexican-American patients requires understanding of cultural differences:

- Some immigrant Mexicans have very little formal education, so medical information may seem very complex and confusing, and they may not understand the implications or need for follow-up care.
- Mexican culture perceives time with more flexibility than American, so if parents need to be present at a particular time, the nurse should specify the exact time (1:30 PM) and explain the reason rather than saying something more vague, such as "after lunch."
- People may appear to be unassertive or unable to make decisions when they are simply showing respect to the nurse by being deferent.
- In traditional families, the males make decisions, so a woman may wait for the father or other males in the family to make decisions about treatment or care.
- Families may choose to use folk medicines instead of Western medical care or may combine the two.
- Children and young women are often sheltered and are taught to be respectful to adults, so they may not express their needs openly.

Middle Eastern Patients

Male/Female Issues

There are considerable cultural differences among Middle Easterners, but religious beliefs about the segregation of males and females are common. It's important to remember that segregating the female is meant to protect her virtue. Female nurses have low status in many countries because they violate this segregation by touching male bodies, so parents may not trust or show respect for the nurse who is caring for their family member. Additionally, male patients may not want to be cared for by female nurses or doctors, and families may be very upset at a female being cared for by a male nurse or physician. When possible, these cultural traditions should be accommodated:

- In Middle Eastern countries, males make decisions, so issues for discussion or decision should be directed to males, such as the father or spouse, and males may be direct in stating what they want, sometimes appearing demanding.
- If a male nurse must care for a female patient, then the family should be advised that personal care (such as bathing) will be done by a female while the medical treatments will be done by the male nurse.

Diet, Language, Families, Medical Care, Grief, and Gift Giving
Caring for Middle Eastern patients requires understanding of cultural differences:

- Families may practice strict dietary restrictions, such as avoiding pork and requiring that animals be killed in a ritual manner, so vegetarian or kosher meals may be required.
- People may have language difficulties requiring a translator, and same-sex translators should be used if at all possible.
- Families may be accompanied by large extended families that want to be kept informed and whom patients consult before decisions are made.
- Most medical care is provided by female relatives, so educating the family about patient care should be directed at females (with female translators if necessary).
- Outward expressions of grief are considered as showing respect for the dead.
- Middle Eastern families often offer gifts to caregivers. Small gifts (candy) should be accepted graciously, but for other gifts, the families should be advised graciously that accepting gifts is against hospital policy.
- Middle Easterners often require less personal space and may stand very close.

Asian Patients

Respect, Disagreement, and Eye Contact
There are considerable differences among different Asian populations, so cultural generalizations may not apply to all, but nurses caring for Asian patients should be aware of common cultural attitudes and behaviors:

- Nurses and doctors are viewed with respect, so traditional Asian families may expect the nurse to remain authoritative and to give directions and may not question, so the nurse should ensure that they understand by having them review material or give demonstrations and should provide explanations clearly, anticipating questions that the family might have but may not articulate.
- Disagreeing is considered impolite. "Yes" may only mean that the person is heard, not that they agree with the person. When asked if they understand, they may indicate that they do even when they clearly do not so as not to offend the nurse.
- Asians may avoid eye contact as an indication of respect. This is especially true of children in relation to adults and younger adults in relation to elders.

Emotions, Illness, Informing The Patient, Non-Traditional Treatments, Language, and Family Dynamics
Caring for Asian patients requires understanding of cultural differences:

- Patients/families may not show outward expressions of feelings/grief, sometimes appearing passive. They also avoid public displays of affection. This does not mean that they don't feel, just that they don't show their feelings.
- Families often hide illness and disabilities from others and may feel ashamed about illness.
- Terminal illness is often hidden from the patient, so families may not want patients to know they are dying or seriously ill.
- Families may use cupping, pinching, or applying pressure to injured areas, and this can leave bruises that may appear as abuse, so when bruises are found, the family should be questioned about alternative therapy before assumptions are made.
- Patients may be treated with traditional herbs.
- Families may need translators because of poor or no English skills.
- In traditional Asian families, males are authoritative and make the decisions.

Clinical inquiry

The ACCN Synergy Model

According to the ACCN Synergy model, clinical inquiry is a continual process of questioning and evaluating practice in order to provide innovative and outstanding care through application of the results of research and experience. Clinical inquiry requires a desire to acquire new knowledge, openness to accepting advice from mentors and other health and allied professionals, competency in identifying clinical problems, and the ability search the literature for research, critical skills to interpret research findings, and to willingness and ability to design and participate in research.

Levels of clinical inquiry include:
- Level 1: This nurse recognizes problems and seeks advice, follows industry standards and guidelines, and seeks further knowledge.
- Level 3: This nurse questions industry standards and guidelines as well as current practice and utilizes research and education to improve patient care.
- Level 5: This nurse is able to deviate from industry standards and guidelines when necessary for the individual patients and utilizes literature review and clinical research to gain knowledge, establish new practices, and improve patient care.

<u>Steps to Evidence-Based Guidelines</u>

Steps to evidence-based practice guidelines include:
- Focus on the topic/methodology: This includes outlining possible interventions/treatments for review, choosing patient populations and settings and determining significant outcomes. Search boundaries (such as types of journals, types of studies, dates of studies) should be determined.
- Evidence review: This includes review of literature, critical analysis of studies, and summarizing of results, including pooled meta-analysis.
- Expert judgment: Recommendations based on personal experience from a number of experts may be utilized, especially if there is inadequate evidence based on review, but this subjective evidence should be explicated acknowledged.

- Policy considerations: This includes cost-effectiveness, access to care, insurance coverage, availability of qualified staff, and legal implications.
- Policy: A written policy must be completed with recommendations. Common practice is to utilize letter guidelines, with "A" the most highly recommended, usually based the quality of supporting evidence.
- Review: The completed policy should be submitted to peers for review and comments before instituting the policy.

Research

Basic Research Concepts
The nurse must be taught and understand the process of critical analysis and know how to conduct a survey of the literature.

Basic research concepts include:
- Survey of valid sources: Information from a juried journal and an anonymous website or personal website are very different sources, and evaluating what constitutes a valid source of data is critical.
- Evaluation of internal and external validity: Internal validity shows a cause and effect relationship between two variables, with the cause occurring before the effect and no intervening variable. External validity occurs when results hold true in different environments and circumstances with different populations.
- Sample selection and sample size: Selection and size can have a huge impact on the results, but a sample that is too small may lack both internal and external validity. Selection may be so narrowly focused that the results can't be generalized to others groups.

Critical Reading of Research Article
There are a number of steps to critical reading to evaluate research:
- Consider the source of the material. If it is in the popular press, it may have little validity compared to something published in a juried journal.
- Review the author's credentials to determine if a person is an expert in the field of study.
- Determine thesis, or the central claim of the research. It should be clearly stated.
- Examine the organization of the article, whether it is based on a particular theory, and the type of methodology used.
- Review the evidence to determine how it is used to support the main points. Look for statistical evidence and sample size to determine if the findings have wide applicability.
- Evaluate the overall article to determine if the information seems credible and useful and should be communicated to administration and/or staff.

Internal And External Validity, Generalizability, and Replication
Many research studies are most concerned with internal validity, adequate unbiased data properly collected and analyzed within the population studied, but studies that determine the efficacy of procedures or treatments, for example, should have external validity as well; that is, the results should be generalizable (true) for similar populations.

Replication of the study with different subjects, researchers, and under different circumstances should produce similar results. For various reasons, some people may be excluded from a study so that instead of randomized subjects, the subjects may be highly selected so when data is compared with another population in which there is less or more selection, results may be different. The selection of subjects, in this case, would interfere with external validity. Part of the design of a study should include considerations of whether or not it should have external validity or whether there is value for the institution based solely on internal validation.

<u>Selection and Information Bias</u>

Selection bias occurs when the method of selecting subjects results in a cohort that is not representative of the target population because of inherent error in design. For example, if all children who develop urinary infections are evaluated per urine culture and sensitivities for microbial resistance, but only those children with clinically-evident infections are included, a number of children with sub-clinical infections may be missed, skewing the results. Selection bias is only a concern when participants in studies are specifically chosen. Many surveillance studies do not involve selection of subjects.

Information bias occurs when there are errors in classification, so an estimate of association is incorrect. Non-differential misclassification occurs when there is similar misclassification of disease or exposure among both those who are diseased/exposed and those who are not. Differential misclassification occurs when there is a differing misclassification of disease or exposure among both those who are diseased/exposed and those who are not.

<u>Hypothesis and Hypothesis Testing</u>

A hypothesis should be generated about the probable cause of the disease/infection based on the information available in laboratory and medical records, epidemiologic study, literature review, and expert opinion. A hypothesis, for example, should include the infective agent, the likely source, and the mode of transmission: "Wound infections with *Staphylococcus aureus* were caused by reuse and inadequate sterilization of single-use irrigation syringes used during wound care in the ICU."

Hypothesis testing includes data analysis, laboratory findings, and outcomes of environmental testing. It usually includes case control studies, with 2-4 controls picked for each case of infection. They may be matched according to age, sex, or other characteristics, but they are not infected at the time they are picked for the study. Cohort studies, whose controls are picked based on having or lacking exposure, may also be instituted. If the hypothesis cannot be supported, then a new hypothesis or different testing methods may be necessary.

Outcomes Evaluation and Evidence-Based Practice

Outcomes evaluation is an important component of evidence-based practice, which involves both internal and external research. All treatments are subjected to review to determine if they produce positive outcomes, and policies and protocols for outcomes evaluation should be in place. Outcomes evaluation includes the following:

- Monitoring over the course of treatment involves careful observation and record keeping that notes progress, with supporting laboratory and radiographic evidence as indicated by condition and treatment.

- Evaluating results includes reviewing records as well as current research to determine if outcomes are within acceptable parameters.
- Sustaining involves continuing treatment, but continuing to monitor and evaluate.
- Improving means to continue the treatment but with additions or modifications in order to improve outcomes.
- Replacing the treatment with a different treatment must be done if outcomes evaluation indicates that current treatment is ineffective.

Qualitative and Quantitative Data

Both qualitative and quantitative data are used for analysis, but the focus is quite different:
- Qualitative data: Data are described verbally or graphically, and the results are subjective, depending upon observers to provide information. Interviews may be used as a tool to gather information, and the researcher's interpretation of data is important. Gathering this type of data can be time-intensive, and it can usually not be generalized to a larger population. This type of information gathering is often useful at the beginning of the design process for data collection.
- Quantitative data: Data are described in terms of numbers within a statistical format. This type of information gathering is done after the design of data collection is outlined, usually in later stages. Tools may include surveys, questionnaires, or other methods of obtaining numerical data. The researcher's role is objective.

Facilitation of Learning

The ACCN Synergy Model

According to the ACCN Synergy model, facilitation of learning is the ability to facilitate learning by patient and family/caregivers as well as other health and allied professionals and community members. Facilitation of learning requires needs assessment and preparation of content that is suited for the receiver in terms of delivery and content. Levels of facilitation of learning include:
- Level 1: This nurse is able to deliver planned educational content that is disease specific but does not have the ability to assess patient readiness to learn or abilities. The patient/family is considered a passive recipient of knowledge.
- Level 3: This nurse is able to individualize treatment according to patient/family needs and has an understanding of different methods of teaching and learning styles. The patient's needs are considered in planning.
- Level 5: This nurse has excellent understanding of teaching methods, learning styles, and assessment for learning readiness and develops an educational plan in cooperation and collaboration with others, including patients, families, and other health and allied professionals.

Bloom's Taxonomy and 3 Types of Learning

Bloom's taxonomy outlines behaviors that are necessary for learning, and this can apply to healthcare.

The theory describes 3 types of learning:

Cognitive (Learning and gaining intellectual skills to master 6 categories of effective learning.)
- Knowledge
- Comprehension
- Application
- Analysis
- Synthesis
    - Evaluation

Affective (Recognizing 5 categories of feelings and values from simple to complex. This is slower to achieve than cognitive learning.)
- Receiving phenomena: Accepting need to learn.
- Responding to phenomena: Taking active part in care.
- Valuing: Understanding value of becoming independent in care.
- Organizing values: Understanding how surgery/treatment has improved life.
- Internalizing values: Accepting condition as part of life, being consistent and self-reliant.

Psychomotor (Mastering 6 motor skills necessary for independence. This follows a progression from simple to complex.)
- Perception: Uses sensory information to learn tasks.
- Set: Shows willingness to perform tasks.
- Guided response: Follows directions.
- Mechanism: Does specific tasks.
- Complex overt response: Displays competence in self-care.
- Adaptation: Modifies procedures as needed.
- Origination: Creatively deals with problems.

Visual-Auditory-Kinesthetic Model of Cognitive Learning

Not all people are aware of their preferred learning style. A range of teaching materials/methods that relates to all 3 learning preferences—visual, auditory, kinesthetic—(and appropriate for different ages) should be available. Part of assessment for teaching involves choosing the right approach based on observation and feedback. Often presenting learners with different options gives a clue to their preferred learning style. Some people have a combined learning style:

Visual learners	Learn best by seeing and reading: Provide written directions, picture guides, or demonstrate procedures. Use charts and diagrams. Provide photos, videos.
Auditory learners	Learn best by listening and talking:Procedures while demonstrating and have learner repeat. Plan extra time to discuss and answer questions. Provide audiotapes.

Kinesthetic learners	Learn best by handling, doing, and practicing: Provide hands-on experience throughout teaching. Encourage handling of supplies/equipment. Allow learner to demonstrate. Minimize instructions and allow person to explore equipment and procedures.

Evaluating the Effectiveness of Education/ Training

Behavior Modification and Compliance Rate

Education, like all interventions, must be evaluated for effectiveness. Two determinants of effectiveness include:

- Behavior modification involves thorough observation and measurement, identifying behavior that needs to be changed and then planning and instituting interventions to modify that behavior. A nurse can use a variety of techniques, including demonstrations of appropriate behavior, reinforcement, and monitoring until new behavior is adopted consistently. This is especially important when longstanding procedures and habits of behavior are changed.
- Compliance rates are often determined by observation, which should be done at intervals and on multiple occasions, but with patients, this may depend on self-reports. Outcomes is another measure of compliance; that is, if education is intended to improve patient health and reduce risk factors and that occurs, it is a good indication that there is compliance. Compliance rates are calculated by determining the number of events/procedures and degree of compliance.

How The Developmental Stage of Learner Affects Teaching and Independent Care

Patients at all developmental stages should be independent in care if at all possible, especially for chronic conditions:

- Infant/toddler: Caregivers provide care; instruction encourages bonding and acceptance.
- Early childhood: Children learn by participation, such as role-playing, simple explanation, and teaching dolls. Children can be independent in some procedures by kindergarten.
- Childhood: By 6, children may be independent in care at school, but supplies should be available and school nurse knowledgeable about care. Children should be completely independent in care by 6th grade. Parents and child should be taught together.
- Adolescence/ young adulthood: The adolescent may be angry and resistive. Extra time and guidance, including visits with other patients, may help. Parents should allow adolescent to be independent in care.

Teaching/Learning

Infants and Toddlers

Almost all teaching is geared toward the parents/caregivers for the child's **first two years**, but during the second year, children's cognitive abilities mature to the point that they have some memory of events (but limited recall), begin to understand the permanence of objects, and can begin to associate cause and effect. Children have short attention spans and are easily distracted. Teaching children at this stage usually involves increasing their acceptance and tolerance of treatment.

Techniques include:
- Interact with the child when he/she feels secure (held by a parent).
- Smile, talk to the child often.
- Use toys, such as dolls and puppets, to demonstrate feelings.
- Read age-appropriate medical stories with pictures to the child.
- Allow the child to handle materials or equipment—such as oxygen masks or dressing material—when possible.
- Demonstrate treatments/procedures on a doll or teddy bear, making a game of it and encouraging the child to play.
- Use repetition and limit teaching periods to 5 minutes.

Early Childhood
From ages 3 to 5, children move from toddlerhood into childhood and fine and gross motor skills improve, allowing children to be more autonomous and independent in personal care. Children can talk and reason, and recall improves, but they have a limited perception of time. They have little understanding of explanations, and they may have magical thinking and fear of pain or injury. Children are more social and interact and play with others, including role-playing. While much teaching is aimed at the parents, the child should be an active participant at this stage:
- Use visual and kinesthetic methods of teaching.
- Limit teaching to 15 minutes but repeat frequently and keep explanations simple.
- Provide tangible rewards (small toys) for participation.
- Connect activities to familiar events (breathing exercises/blowing up balloons).
- Encourage child to manipulate equipment.
- Use special medical dolls to show body parts, etc.
- Use storybooks.
- Allow child to make some decisions (play with medical doll or read book).

Childhood
From ages 6 to 11, children at this stage vary widely in physical maturity, but they have increasing control of fine and gross motor skills, are receptive to learning, can question and reason. Thinking remains literal rather than abstract. Concentration improves with age, and older children have a better understanding of their body and body systems. They are used to structured education. Children interact with peers and fear being different or ill. Teaching is aimed at the child with the parents as support (especially in later childhood):
- Allow children to assume responsibility for much of their care.
- Limit teaching to about 30 minutes and allow time for the child to absorb/study material.
- Provide age-specific materials, such as Kid Cards (medicine information cards).
- Use a variety of teaching materials, including pictures, diagrams, and illustrations.
- Use analogies (A CT is like a giant camera).
- Use one-on-one or group instruction as appropriate.
- Tell children about treatments/procedures in advance.
- Provide support and encourage questions and participation.

Adolescents
Adolescents vary widely in both physical and emotional maturity, but they have good reasoning and abstract thinking skills, understand cause and effect, and have good motor

skills, but may engage in risk-taking behaviors and may have difficulty dealing with illness and poor compliance with treatments. They are very conscious of their body image and have a strong need to belong to a peer group while rebelling against authority. They wish to be independent and need privacy and confidentiality. Teaching is aimed at allowing the adolescent to be independent in care:

- Use one-on-one (for confidential teaching) or peer group instruction/discussion as appropriate.
- Supplement instruction with audiovisual materials, computer-generated instruction, models, diagrams, illustrations, and written instructions, focusing on learning style and learning preferences.
- Allow the adolescent to maintain as much control over learning as possible.
- Provide options from which the adolescent can choose.
- Be patient, respectful, and tactful.
- Provide reasons for everything.
- Avoid conflict and direct confrontation, but suggest alternatives.

Kid Cards

One of the challenges to facilitating learning in children is to teach them about their medications. Kid Cards are medicine information cards that present important details about the medication in language that is age-appropriate and often with pictures or illustrations. Information on a Kid Card may include:

Acetaminophen
This medicine is also called Tylenol®

Why am I taking Tylenol?
You have to take this medicine so you can exercise your arm.
It helps to keep your arm from hurting.

How do I take Tylenol?
It is a chewable tablet (about the size of an M&M).
You need to chew 5 tablets with breakfast and 5 with lunch and 5 with dinner for 4 or 5 days.
You can stop taking Tylenol when your arm stops hurting.

What might happen if I take Tylenol?
Most kids don't have any bad effects from taking Tylenol.
If you get a rash, start itching, or feel sick to your stomach, tell your mom right away so she can call the doctor.

The Use of Play to Facilitate Learning

Play can be a useful tool to help children deal with physical and emotional problems related to their illness. Allowing children to play with medical equipment under supervision can allay some of their fears and help them to understand. Needle play, in which the child gives "shots" to a doll (with safe plastic syringes) can help them to express feelings about repeated blood draws or injections. Providing dolls and puppets and engaging in play may encourage the child to express anxiety and fear through "talking" for the toy. There are a number of specialty dolls, such as dolls with removable parts to show internal organs and Shadow Buddies®, which are dolls that are commercially available (custom-made) to show the effects of different illnesses or surgeries. For example, a doll with thinning hair may show the effects of chemotherapy. Other dolls have stomas and colostomy bags. Drawing also may encourage the child to express feelings.

Secret Key #1 - Time is Your Greatest Enemy

Pace Yourself

Wear a watch. At the beginning of the test, check the time (or start a chronometer on your watch to count the minutes), and check the time after every few questions to make sure you are "on schedule."

If you are forced to speed up, do it efficiently. Usually one or more answer choices can be eliminated without too much difficulty. Above all, don't panic. Don't speed up and just begin guessing at random choices. By pacing yourself, and continually monitoring your progress against your watch, you will always know exactly how far ahead or behind you are with your available time. If you find that you are one minute behind on the test, don't skip one question without spending any time on it, just to catch back up. Take 15 fewer seconds on the next four questions, and after four questions you'll have caught back up. Once you catch back up, you can continue working each problem at your normal pace.

Furthermore, don't dwell on the problems that you were rushed on. If a problem was taking up too much time and you made a hurried guess, it must be difficult. The difficult questions are the ones you are most likely to miss anyway, so it isn't a big loss. It is better to end with more time than you need than to run out of time.

Lastly, sometimes it is beneficial to slow down if you are constantly getting ahead of time. You are always more likely to catch a careless mistake by working more slowly than quickly, and among very high-scoring test takers (those who are likely to have lots of time left over), careless errors affect the score more than mastery of material.

Secret Key #2 - Guessing is not Guesswork

You probably know that guessing is a good idea - unlike other standardized tests, there is no penalty for getting a wrong answer. Even if you have no idea about a question, you still have a 20-25% chance of getting it right.

Most test takers do not understand the impact that proper guessing can have on their score. Unless you score extremely high, guessing will significantly contribute to your final score.

Monkeys Take the Test

What most test takers don't realize is that to insure that 20-25% chance, you have to guess randomly. If you put 20 monkeys in a room to take this test, assuming they answered once per question and behaved themselves, on average they would get 20-25% of the questions correct. Put 20 test takers in the room, and the average will be much lower among guessed questions. Why?

1. The test writers intentionally write deceptive answer choices that "look" right. A test taker has no idea about a question, so picks the "best looking" answer, which is often wrong. The monkey has no idea what looks good and what doesn't, so will consistently be lucky about 20-25% of the time.
2. Test takers will eliminate answer choices from the guessing pool based on a hunch or intuition. Simple but correct answers often get excluded, leaving a 0% chance of being correct. The monkey has no clue, and often gets lucky with the best choice.

This is why the process of elimination endorsed by most test courses is flawed and detrimental to your performance- test takers don't guess, they make an ignorant stab in the dark that is usually worse than random.

$5 Challenge

Let me introduce one of the most valuable ideas of this course- the $5 challenge:

You only mark your "best guess" if you are willing to bet $5 on it.
You only eliminate choices from guessing if you are willing to bet $5 on it.

Why $5? Five dollars is an amount of money that is small yet not insignificant, and can really add up fast (20 questions could cost you $100). Likewise, each answer choice on one question of the test will have a small impact on your overall score, but it can really add up to a lot of points in the end.

The process of elimination IS valuable. The following shows your chance of guessing it right:

If you eliminate wrong answer choices until only this many remain:	Chance of getting it correct:
1	100%
2	50%
3	33%

However, if you accidentally eliminate the right answer or go on a hunch for an incorrect answer, your chances drop dramatically: to 0%. By guessing among all the answer choices, you are GUARANTEED to have a shot at the right answer.

That's why the $5 test is so valuable- if you give up the advantage and safety of a pure guess, it had better be worth the risk.

What we still haven't covered is how to be sure that whatever guess you make is truly random. Here's the easiest way:

Always pick the first answer choice among those remaining.

Such a technique means that you have decided, **before you see a single test question**, exactly how you are going to guess- and since the order of choices tells you nothing about which one is correct, this guessing technique is perfectly random.

This section is not meant to scare you away from making educated guesses or eliminating choices- you just need to define when a choice is worth eliminating. The $5 test, along with a pre-defined random guessing strategy, is the best way to make sure you reap all of the benefits of guessing.

Secret Key #3 - Practice Smarter, Not Harder

Many test takers delay the test preparation process because they dread the awful amounts of practice time they think necessary to succeed on the test. We have refined an effective method that will take you only a fraction of the time.

There are a number of "obstacles" in your way to succeed. Among these are answering questions, finishing in time, and mastering test-taking strategies. All must be executed on the day of the test at peak performance, or your score will suffer. The test is a mental marathon that has a large impact on your future.

Just like a marathon runner, it is important to work your way up to the full challenge. So first you just worry about questions, and then time, and finally strategy:

Success Strategy

1. Find a good source for practice tests.
2. If you are willing to make a larger time investment, consider using more than one study guide- often the different approaches of multiple authors will help you "get" difficult concepts.
3. Take a practice test with no time constraints, with all study helps "open book." Take your time with questions and focus on applying strategies.
4. Take a practice test with time constraints, with all guides "open book."
5. Take a final practice test with no open material and time limits

If you have time to take more practice tests, just repeat step 5. By gradually exposing yourself to the full rigors of the test environment, you will condition your mind to the stress of test day and maximize your success.

Secret Key #4 - Prepare, Don't Procrastinate

Let me state an obvious fact: if you take the test three times, you will get three different scores. This is due to the way you feel on test day, the level of preparedness you have, and, despite the test writers' claims to the contrary, some tests WILL be easier for you than others.

Since your future depends so much on your score, you should maximize your chances of success. In order to maximize the likelihood of success, you've got to prepare in advance. This means taking practice tests and spending time learning the information and test taking strategies you will need to succeed.

Never take the test as a "practice" test, expecting that you can just take it again if you need to. Feel free to take sample tests on your own, but when you go to take the official test, be prepared, be focused, and do your best the first time!

Secret Key #5 - Test Yourself

Everyone knows that time is money. There is no need to spend too much of your time or too little of your time preparing for the test. You should only spend as much of your precious time preparing as is necessary for you to get the score you need.

Once you have taken a practice test under real conditions of time constraints, then you will know if you are ready for the test or not.

If you have scored extremely high the first time that you take the practice test, then there is not much point in spending countless hours studying. You are already there.

Benchmark your abilities by retaking practice tests and seeing how much you have improved. Once you score high enough to guarantee success, then you are ready.

If you have scored well below where you need, then knuckle down and begin studying in earnest. Check your improvement regularly through the use of practice tests under real conditions. Above all, don't worry, panic, or give up. The key is perseverance!

Then, when you go to take the test, remain confident and remember how well you did on the practice tests. If you can score high enough on a practice test, then you can do the same on the real thing.

General Strategies

The most important thing you can do is to ignore your fears and jump into the test immediately- do not be overwhelmed by any strange-sounding terms. You have to jump into the test like jumping into a pool- all at once is the easiest way.

Make Predictions
As you read and understand the question, try to guess what the answer will be. Remember that several of the answer choices are wrong, and once you begin reading them, your mind will immediately become cluttered with answer choices designed to throw you off. Your mind is typically the most focused immediately after you have read the question and digested its contents. If you can, try to predict what the correct answer will be. You may be

surprised at what you can predict.

Quickly scan the choices and see if your prediction is in the listed answer choices. If it is, then you can be quite confident that you have the right answer. It still won't hurt to check the other answer choices, but most of the time, you've got it!

Answer the Question
It may seem obvious to only pick answer choices that answer the question, but the test writers can create some excellent answer choices that are wrong. Don't pick an answer just because it sounds right, or you believe it to be true. It MUST answer the question. Once you've made your selection, always go back and check it against the question and make sure that you didn't misread the question, and the answer choice does answer the question posed.

Benchmark
After you read the first answer choice, decide if you think it sounds correct or not. If it doesn't, move on to the next answer choice. If it does, mentally mark that answer choice. This doesn't mean that you've definitely selected it as your answer choice, it just means that it's the best you've seen thus far. Go ahead and read the next choice. If the next choice is worse than the one you've already selected, keep going to the next answer choice. If the next choice is better than the choice you've already selected, mentally mark the new answer choice as your best guess.

The first answer choice that you select becomes your standard. Every other answer choice must be benchmarked against that standard. That choice is correct until proven otherwise by another answer choice beating it out. Once you've decided that no other answer choice seems as good, do one final check to ensure that your answer choice answers the question posed.

Valid Information
Don't discount any of the information provided in the question. Every piece of information may be necessary to determine the correct answer. None of the information in the question is there to throw you off (while the answer choices will certainly have information to throw you off). If two seemingly unrelated topics are discussed, don't ignore either. You can be confident there is a relationship, or it wouldn't be included in the question, and you are probably going to have to determine what is that relationship to find the answer.

Avoid "Fact Traps"
Don't get distracted by a choice that is factually true. Your search is for the answer that answers the question. Stay focused and don't fall for an answer that is true but incorrect. Always go back to the question and make sure you're choosing an answer that actually answers the question and is not just a true statement. An answer can be factually correct, but it MUST answer the question asked. Additionally, two answers can both be seemingly correct, so be sure to read all of the answer choices, and make sure that you get the one that BEST answers the question.

Milk the Question
Some of the questions may throw you completely off. They might deal with a subject you have not been exposed to, or one that you haven't reviewed in years. While your lack of knowledge about the subject will be a hindrance, the question itself can give you many clues that will help you find the correct answer. Read the question carefully and look for clues.

Watch particularly for adjectives and nouns describing difficult terms or words that you don't recognize. Regardless of if you completely understand a word or not, replacing it with a synonym either provided or one you more familiar with may help you to understand what the questions are asking. Rather than wracking your mind about specific detailed information concerning a difficult term or word, try to use mental substitutes that are easier to understand.

The Trap of Familiarity

Don't just choose a word because you recognize it. On difficult questions, you may not recognize a number of words in the answer choices. The test writers don't put "make-believe" words on the test; so don't think that just because you only recognize all the words in one answer choice means that answer choice must be correct. If you only recognize words in one answer choice, then focus on that one. Is it correct? Try your best to determine if it is correct. If it is, that is great, but if it doesn't, eliminate it. Each word and answer choice you eliminate increases your chances of getting the question correct, even if you then have to guess among the unfamiliar choices.

Eliminate Answers

Eliminate choices as soon as you realize they are wrong. But be careful! Make sure you consider all of the possible answer choices. Just because one appears right, doesn't mean that the next one won't be even better! The test writers will usually put more than one good answer choice for every question, so read all of them. Don't worry if you are stuck between two that seem right. By getting down to just two remaining possible choices, your odds are now 50/50. Rather than wasting too much time, play the odds. You are guessing, but guessing wisely, because you've been able to knock out some of the answer choices that you know are wrong. If you are eliminating choices and realize that the last answer choice you are left with is also obviously wrong, don't panic. Start over and consider each choice again. There may easily be something that you missed the first time and will realize on the second pass.

Tough Questions

If you are stumped on a problem or it appears too hard or too difficult, don't waste time. Move on! Remember though, if you can quickly check for obviously incorrect answer choices, your chances of guessing correctly are greatly improved. Before you completely give up, at least try to knock out a couple of possible answers. Eliminate what you can and then guess at the remaining answer choices before moving on.

Brainstorm

If you get stuck on a difficult question, spend a few seconds quickly brainstorming. Run through the complete list of possible answer choices. Look at each choice and ask yourself, "Could this answer the question satisfactorily?" Go through each answer choice and consider it independently of the other. By systematically going through all possibilities, you may find something that you would otherwise overlook. Remember that when you get stuck, it's important to try to keep moving.

Read Carefully

Understand the problem. Read the question and answer choices carefully. Don't miss the question because you misread the terms. You have plenty of time to read each question thoroughly and make sure you understand what is being asked. Yet a happy medium must be attained, so don't waste too much time. You must read carefully, but efficiently.

Face Value

When in doubt, use common sense. Always accept the situation in the problem at face value. Don't read too much into it. These problems will not require you to make huge leaps of logic. The test writers aren't trying to throw you off with a cheap trick. If you have to go beyond creativity and make a leap of logic in order to have an answer choice answer the question, then you should look at the other answer choices. Don't overcomplicate the problem by creating theoretical relationships or explanations that will warp time or space. These are normal problems rooted in reality. It's just that the applicable relationship or explanation may not be readily apparent and you have to figure things out. Use your common sense to interpret anything that isn't clear.

Prefixes

If you're having trouble with a word in the question or answer choices, try dissecting it. Take advantage of every clue that the word might include. Prefixes and suffixes can be a huge help. Usually they allow you to determine a basic meaning. Pre- means before, post- means after, pro - is positive, de- is negative. From these prefixes and suffixes, you can get an idea of the general meaning of the word and try to put it into context. Beware though of any traps. Just because con is the opposite of pro, doesn't necessarily mean congress is the opposite of progress!

Hedge Phrases

Watch out for critical "hedge" phrases, such as likely, may, can, will often, sometimes, often, almost, mostly, usually, generally, rarely, sometimes. Question writers insert these hedge phrases to cover every possibility. Often an answer choice will be wrong simply because it leaves no room for exception. Avoid answer choices that have definitive words like "exactly," and "always".

Switchback Words

Stay alert for "switchbacks". These are the words and phrases frequently used to alert you to shifts in thought. The most common switchback word is "but". Others include although, however, nevertheless, on the other hand, even though, while, in spite of, despite, regardless of.

New Information

Correct answer choices will rarely have completely new information included. Answer choices typically are straightforward reflections of the material asked about and will directly relate to the question. If a new piece of information is included in an answer choice that doesn't even seem to relate to the topic being asked about, then that answer choice is likely incorrect. All of the information needed to answer the question is usually provided for you, and so you should not have to make guesses that are unsupported or choose answer choices that require unknown information that cannot be reasoned on its own.

Time Management

On technical questions, don't get lost on the technical terms. Don't spend too much time on any one question. If you don't know what a term means, then since you don't have a dictionary, odds are you aren't going to get much further. You should immediately recognize terms as whether or not you know them. If you don't, work with the other clues that you have, the other answer choices and terms provided, but don't waste too much time trying to figure out a difficult term.

Contextual Clues

Look for contextual clues. An answer can be right but not correct. The contextual clues will help you find the answer that is most right and is correct. Understand the context in which a phrase or statement is made. This will help you make important distinctions.

Don't Panic

Panicking will not answer any questions for you. Therefore, it isn't helpful. When you first see the question, if your mind goes blank, take a deep breath. Force yourself to mechanically go through the steps of solving the problem and using the strategies you've learned.

Pace Yourself

Don't get clock fever. It's easy to be overwhelmed when you're looking at a page full of questions, your mind is full of random thoughts and feeling confused, and the clock is ticking down faster than you would like. Calm down and maintain the pace that you have set for yourself. As long as you are on track by monitoring your pace, you are guaranteed to have enough time for yourself. When you get to the last few minutes of the test, it may seem like you won't have enough time left, but if you only have as many questions as you should have left at that point, then you're right on track!

Answer Selection

The best way to pick an answer choice is to eliminate all of those that are wrong, until only one is left and confirm that is the correct answer. Sometimes though, an answer choice may immediately look right. Be careful! Take a second to make sure that the other choices are not equally obvious. Don't make a hasty mistake. There are only two times that you should stop before checking other answers. First is when you are positive that the answer choice you have selected is correct. Second is when time is almost out and you have to make a quick guess!

Check Your Work

Since you will probably not know every term listed and the answer to every question, it is important that you get credit for the ones that you do know. Don't miss any questions through careless mistakes. If at all possible, try to take a second to look back over your answer selection and make sure you've selected the correct answer choice and haven't made a costly careless mistake (such as marking an answer choice that you didn't mean to mark). This quick double check should more than pay for itself in caught mistakes for the time it costs.

Beware of Directly Quoted Answers

Sometimes an answer choice will repeat word for word a portion of the question or reference section. However, beware of such exact duplication – it may be a trap! More than likely, the correct choice will paraphrase or summarize a point, rather than being exactly the same wording.

Slang

Scientific sounding answers are better than slang ones. An answer choice that begins "To compare the outcomes..." is much more likely to be correct than one that begins "Because some people insisted..."

Extreme Statements

Avoid wild answers that throw out highly controversial ideas that are proclaimed as established fact. An answer choice that states the "process should be used in certain situations, if…" is much more likely to be correct than one that states the "process should be discontinued completely." The first is a calm rational statement and doesn't even make a definitive, uncompromising stance, using a hedge word "if" to provide wiggle room, whereas the second choice is a radical idea and far more extreme.

Answer Choice Families

When you have two or more answer choices that are direct opposites or parallels, one of them is usually the correct answer. For instance, if one answer choice states "x increases" and another answer choice states "x decreases" or "y increases," then those two or three answer choices are very similar in construction and fall into the same family of answer choices. A family of answer choices is when two or three answer choices are very similar in construction, and yet often have a directly opposite meaning. Usually the correct answer choice will be in that family of answer choices. The "odd man out" or answer choice that doesn't seem to fit the parallel construction of the other answer choices is more likely to be incorrect.

Special Report: What Your Test Score Will Tell You About Your IQ

Did you know that most standardized tests correlate very strongly with IQ? In fact, your general intelligence is a better predictor of your success than any other factor, and most tests intentionally measure this trait to some degree to ensure that those selected by the test are truly qualified for the test's purposes.

Before we can delve into the relation between your test score and IQ, I will first have to explain what exactly is IQ. Here's the formula:

Your IQ = 100 + (Number of standard deviations below or above the average)*15

Now, let's define standard deviations by using an example. If we have 5 people with 5 different heights, then first we calculate the average. Let's say the average was 65 inches. The standard deviation is the "average distance" away from the average of each of the members. It is a direct measure of variability - if the 5 people included Jackie Chan and Shaquille O'Neal, obviously there's a lot more variability in that group than a group of 5 sisters who are all within 6 inches in height of each other. The standard deviation uses a number to characterize the average range of difference within a group.

A convenient feature of most groups is that they have a "normal" distribution- makes sense that most things would be normal, right? Without getting into a bunch of statistical mumbo-jumbo, you just need to know that if you know the average of the group and the standard deviation, you can successfully predict someone's percentile rank in the group.

Confused? Let me give you an example. If instead of 5 people's heights, we had 100 people, we could figure out their rank in height JUST by knowing the average, standard deviation, and their height. We wouldn't need to know each person's height and manually rank them, we could just predict their rank based on three numbers.

What this means is that you can take your PERCENTILE rank that is often given with your test and relate this to your RELATIVE IQ of people taking the test - that is, your IQ relative to the people taking the test. Obviously, there's no way to know your actual IQ because the people taking a standardized test are usually not very good samples of the general population- many of those with extremely low IQ's never achieve a level of success or competency necessary to complete a typical standardized test. In fact, professional psychologists who measure IQ actually have to use non-written tests that can fairly measure the IQ of those not able to complete a traditional test.

The bottom line is to not take your test score too seriously, but it is fun to compute your "relative IQ" among the people who took the test with you. I've done the calculations below. Just look up your percentile rank in the left and then you'll see your "relative IQ" for your test in the right hand column-

Percentile Rank	Your Relative IQ		Percentile Rank	Your Relative IQ
99	135		59	103
98	131		58	103
97	128		57	103
96	126		56	102
95	125		55	102
94	123		54	102
93	122		53	101
92	121		52	101
91	120		51	100
90	119		50	100
89	118		49	100
88	118		48	99
87	117		47	99
86	116		46	98
85	116		45	98
84	115		44	98
83	114		43	97
82	114		42	97
81	113		41	97
80	113		40	96
79	112		39	96
78	112		38	95
77	111		37	95
76	111		36	95
75	110		35	94
74	110		34	94
73	109		33	93
72	109		32	93
71	108		31	93
70	108		30	92
69	107		29	92
68	107		28	91
67	107		27	91
66	106		26	90
65	106		25	90
64	105		24	89
63	105		23	89
62	105		22	88
61	104		21	88
60	104		20	87

Special Report: How to Overcome Test Anxiety

The very nature of tests caters to some level of anxiety, nervousness or tension, just as we feel for any important event that occurs in our lives. A little bit of anxiety or nervousness can be a good thing. It helps us with motivation, and makes achievement just that much sweeter. However, too much anxiety can be a problem; especially if it hinders our ability to function and perform.

"Test anxiety," is the term that refers to the emotional reactions that some test-takers experience when faced with a test or exam. Having a fear of testing and exams is based upon a rational fear, since the test-taker's performance can shape the course of an academic career. Nevertheless, experiencing excessive fear of examinations will only interfere with the test-takers ability to perform, and his/her chances to be successful.

There are a large variety of causes that can contribute to the development and sensation of test anxiety. These include, but are not limited to lack of performance and worrying about issues surrounding the test.

Lack of Preparation

Lack of preparation can be identified by the following behaviors or situations:

Not scheduling enough time to study, and therefore cramming the night before the test or exam
Managing time poorly, to create the sensation that there is not enough time to do everything
Failing to organize the text information in advance, so that the study material consists of the entire text and not simply the pertinent information
Poor overall studying habits

Worrying, on the other hand, can be related to both the test taker, or many other factors around him/her that will be affected by the results of the test. These include worrying about:

Previous performances on similar exams, or exams in general
How friends and other students are achieving
The negative consequences that will result from a poor grade or failure

There are three primary elements to test anxiety. Physical components, which involve the same typical bodily reactions as those to acute anxiety (to be discussed below). Emotional factors have to do with fear or panic. Mental or cognitive issues concerning attention spans and memory abilities.

Physical Signals

There are many different symptoms of test anxiety, and these are not limited to mental and emotional strain. Frequently there are a range of physical signals that will let a test taker know that he/she is suffering from test anxiety. These bodily changes can include the following:

Perspiring
Sweaty palms
Wet, trembling hands
Nausea
Dry mouth
A knot in the stomach
Headache
Faintness
Muscle tension
Aching shoulders, back and neck
Rapid heart beat
Feeling too hot/cold

To recognize the sensation of test anxiety, a test-taker should monitor him/herself for the following sensations:

The physical distress symptoms as listed above
Emotional sensitivity, expressing emotional feelings such as the need to cry or laugh too much, or a sensation of anger or helplessness
A decreased ability to think, causing the test-taker to blank out or have racing thoughts that are hard to organize or control.

Though most students will feel some level of anxiety when faced with a test or exam, the majority can cope with that anxiety and maintain it at a manageable level. However, those who cannot are faced with a very real and very serious condition, which can and should be controlled for the immeasurable benefit of this sufferer.

Naturally, these sensations lead to negative results for the testing experience. The most common effects of test anxiety have to do with nervousness and mental blocking.

Nervousness

Nervousness can appear in several different levels:

The test-taker's difficulty, or even inability to read and understand the questions on the test
The difficulty or inability to organize thoughts to a coherent form
The difficulty or inability to recall key words and concepts relating to the testing questions (especially essays)

The receipt of poor grades on a test, though the test material was well known by the test taker

Conversely, a person may also experience mental blocking, which involves:

Blanking out on test questions
Only remembering the correct answers to the questions when the test has already finished.

Fortunately for test anxiety sufferers, beating these feelings, to a large degree, has to do with proper preparation. When a test taker has a feeling of preparedness, then anxiety will be dramatically lessened.

The first step to resolving anxiety issues is to distinguish which of the two types of anxiety are being suffered. If the anxiety is a direct result of a lack of preparation, this should be considered a normal reaction, and the anxiety level (as opposed to the test results) shouldn't be anything to worry about. However, if, when adequately prepared, the test-taker still panics, blanks out, or seems to overreact, this is not a fully rational reaction. While this can be considered normal too, there are many ways to combat and overcome these effects.

Remember that anxiety cannot be entirely eliminated, however, there are ways to minimize it, to make the anxiety easier to manage. Preparation is one of the best ways to minimize test anxiety. Therefore the following techniques are wise in order to best fight off any anxiety that may want to build.

To begin with, try to avoid cramming before a test, whenever it is possible. By trying to memorize an entire term's worth of information in one day, you'll be shocking your system, and not giving yourself a very good chance to absorb the information. This is an easy path to anxiety, so for those who suffer from test anxiety, cramming should not even be considered an option.

Instead of cramming, work throughout the semester to combine all of the material which is presented throughout the semester, and work on it gradually as the course goes by, making sure to master the main concepts first, leaving minor details for a week or so before the test.

To study for the upcoming exam, be sure to pose questions that may be on the examination, to gauge the ability to answer them by integrating the ideas from your texts, notes and lectures, as well as any supplementary readings.

If it is truly impossible to cover all of the information that was covered in that particular term, concentrate on the most important portions, that can be covered very well. Learn these concepts as best as possible, so that when the test comes, a goal can be made to use these concepts as presentations of your knowledge.

In addition to study habits, changes in attitude are critical to beating a struggle with test anxiety. In fact, an improvement of the perspective over the entire test-taking experience can actually help a test taker to enjoy studying and therefore improve the overall experience. Be certain not to overemphasize the significance of the grade - know that the result of the test is neither a reflection of self worth, nor is it a measure of intelligence; one grade will not predict a person's future success.

To improve an overall testing outlook, the following steps should be tried:

Keeping in mind that the most reasonable expectation for taking a test is to expect to try to demonstrate as much of what you know as you possibly can.
Reminding ourselves that a test is only one test; this is not the only one, and there will be others.
The thought of thinking of oneself in an irrational, all-or-nothing term should be avoided at all costs.
A reward should be designated for after the test, so there's something to look forward to. Whether it be going to a movie, going out to eat, or simply visiting friends, schedule it in advance, and do it no matter what result is expected on the exam.

Test-takers should also keep in mind that the basics are some of the most important things, even beyond anti-anxiety techniques and studying. Never neglect the basic social, emotional and biological needs, in order to try to absorb information. In order to best achieve, these three factors must be held as just as important as the studying itself.

Study Steps

Remember the following important steps for studying:

Maintain healthy nutrition and exercise habits. Continue both your recreational activities and social pass times. These both contribute to your physical and emotional well being.
Be certain to get a good amount of sleep, especially the night before the test, because when you're overtired you are not able to perform to the best of your best ability.
Keep the studying pace to a moderate level by taking breaks when they are needed, and varying the work whenever possible, to keep the mind fresh instead of getting bored. When enough studying has been done that all the material that can be learned has been learned, and the test taker is prepared for the test, stop studying and do something relaxing such as listening to music, watching a movie, or taking a warm bubble bath.

There are also many other techniques to minimize the uneasiness or apprehension that is experienced along with test anxiety before, during, or even after the examination. In fact, there are a great deal of things that can be done to stop anxiety from interfering with lifestyle and performance. Again, remember that anxiety will not be eliminated entirely, and it shouldn't be. Otherwise that "up" feeling for exams would not exist, and most of us depend on that sensation to perform better than usual. However, this anxiety has to be at a level that is manageable.

Of course, as we have just discussed, being prepared for the exam is half the battle right away. Attending all classes, finding out what knowledge will be expected on the exam, and knowing the exam schedules are easy steps to lowering anxiety. Keeping up with work will remove the need to cram, and efficient study habits will eliminate wasted time. Studying should be done in an ideal location for concentration, so that it is simple to become interested in the material and give it complete attention. A method such as SQ3R (Survey, Question, Read, Recite, Review) is a wonderful key to follow to make sure that the study habits are as effective as possible, especially in the case of learning from a textbook. Flashcards are great techniques for memorization. Learning to take good notes will mean that notes will be full of useful information, so that less sifting will need to be done to seek out what is pertinent for studying. Reviewing notes after class and then again on occasion will keep the information fresh in the mind. From notes that have been taken summary sheets and outlines can be made for simpler reviewing.

A study group can also be a very motivational and helpful place to study, as there will be a sharing of ideas, all of the minds can work together, to make sure that everyone understands, and the studying will be made more interesting because it will be a social occasion.

Basically, though, as long as the test-taker remains organized and self confident, with efficient study habits, less time will need to be spent studying, and higher grades will be achieved.

To become self confident, there are many useful steps. The first of these is "self talk." It has been shown through extensive research, that self-talk for students who suffer from test anxiety, should be well monitored, in order to make sure that it contributes to self confidence as opposed to sinking the student. Frequently the self talk of test-anxious students is negative or self-defeating, thinking that everyone else is smarter and faster, that they always mess up, and that if they don't do well, they'll fail the entire course. It is important to decreasing anxiety that awareness is made of self talk. Try writing any negative self thoughts and then disputing them with a positive statement instead. Begin self-encouragement as though it was a friend speaking. Repeat positive statements to help reprogram the mind to believing in successes instead of failures.

Helpful Techniques

Other extremely helpful techniques include:

Self-visualization of doing well and reaching goals
While aiming for an "A" level of understanding, don't try to "overprotect" by setting your expectations lower. This will only convince the mind to stop studying in order to meet the lower expectations.
Don't make comparisons with the results or habits of other students. These are individual factors, and different things work for different people, causing different results.
Strive to become an expert in learning what works well, and what can be done in order to improve. Consider collecting this data in a journal.
Create rewards for after studying instead of doing things before studying that will only turn into avoidance behaviors.
Make a practice of relaxing - by using methods such as progressive relaxation, self-hypnosis, guided imagery, etc - in order to make relaxation an automatic sensation.

Work on creating a state of relaxed concentration so that concentrating will take on the focus of the mind, so that none will be wasted on worrying.
Take good care of the physical self by eating well and getting enough sleep.
Plan in time for exercise and stick to this plan.

Beyond these techniques, there are other methods to be used before, during and after the test that will help the test-taker perform well in addition to overcoming anxiety.

Before the exam comes the academic preparation. This involves establishing a study schedule and beginning at least one week before the actual date of the test. By doing this, the anxiety of not having enough time to study for the test will be automatically eliminated. Moreover, this will make the studying a much more effective experience, ensuring that the learning will be an easier process. This relieves much undue pressure on the test-taker.

Summary sheets, note cards, and flash cards with the main concepts and examples of these main concepts should be prepared in advance of the actual studying time. A topic should never be eliminated from this process. By omitting a topic because it isn't expected to be on the test is only setting up the test-taker for anxiety should it actually appear on the exam. Utilize the course syllabus for laying out the topics that should be studied. Carefully go over the notes that were made in class, paying special attention to any of the issues that the professor took special care to emphasize while lecturing in class. In the textbooks, use the chapter review, or if possible, the chapter tests, to begin your review.

It may even be possible to ask the instructor what information will be covered on the exam, or what the format of the exam will be (for example, multiple choice, essay, free form, true-false). Additionally, see if it is possible to find out how many questions will be on the test. If a review sheet or sample test has been offered by the professor, make good use of it, above anything else, for the preparation for the test. Another great resource for getting to know the examination is reviewing tests from previous semesters. Use these tests to review, and aim to achieve a 100% score on each of the possible topics. With a few exceptions, the goal that you set for yourself is the highest one that you will reach.

Take all of the questions that were assigned as homework, and rework them to any other possible course material. The more problems reworked, the more skill and confidence will form as a result. When forming the solution to a problem, write out each of the steps. Don't simply do head work. By doing as many steps on paper as possible, much clarification and therefore confidence will be formed. Do this with as many homework problems as possible, before checking the answers. By checking the answer after each problem, a reinforcement will exist, that will not be on the exam. Study situations should be as exam-like as possible, to prime the test-taker's system for the experience. By waiting to check the answers at the end, a psychological advantage will be formed, to decrease the stress factor.

Another fantastic reason for not cramming is the avoidance of confusion in concepts, especially when it comes to mathematics. 8-10 hours of study will become one hundred percent more effective if it is spread out over a week or at least several days, instead of doing it all in one sitting. Recognize that the human brain requires time in order to assimilate new material, so frequent breaks and a span of study time over several days will be much more beneficial.

Additionally, don't study right up until the point of the exam. Studying should stop a minimum of one hour before the exam begins. This allows the brain to rest and put things in their proper order. This will also provide the time to become as relaxed as possible when going into the examination room. The test-taker will also have time to eat well and eat sensibly. Know that the brain needs food as much as the rest of the body. With enough food and enough sleep, as well as a relaxed attitude, the body and the mind are primed for success.

Avoid any anxious classmates who are talking about the exam. These students only spread anxiety, and are not worth sharing the anxious sentimentalities.

Before the test also involves creating a positive attitude, so mental preparation should also be a point of concentration. There are many keys to creating a positive attitude. Should fears become rushing in, make a visualization of taking the exam, doing well, and seeing an A written on the paper. Write out a list of affirmations that will bring a feeling of confidence, such as "I am doing well in my English class," "I studied well and know my material," "I enjoy this class." Even if the affirmations aren't believed at first, it sends a positive message to the subconscious which will result in an alteration of the overall belief system, which is the system that creates reality.

If a sensation of panic begins, work with the fear and imagine the very worst! Work through the entire scenario of not passing the test, failing the entire course, and dropping out of school, followed by not getting a job, and pushing a shopping cart through the dark alley where you'll live. This will place things into perspective! Then, practice deep breathing and create a visualization of the opposite situation - achieving an "A" on the exam, passing the entire course, receiving the degree at a graduation ceremony.

On the day of the test, there are many things to be done to ensure the best results, as well as the most calm outlook. The following stages are suggested in order to maximize test-taking potential:

Begin the examination day with a moderate breakfast, and avoid any coffee or beverages with caffeine if the test taker is prone to jitters. Even people who are used to managing caffeine can feel jittery or light-headed when it is taken on a test day.
Attempt to do something that is relaxing before the examination begins. As last minute cramming clouds the mastering of overall concepts, it is better to use this time to create a calming outlook.
Be certain to arrive at the test location well in advance, in order to provide time to select a location that is away from doors, windows and other distractions, as well as giving enough time to relax before the test begins.
Keep away from anxiety generating classmates who will upset the sensation of stability and relaxation that is being attempted before the exam.
Should the waiting period before the exam begins cause anxiety, create a self-distraction by reading a light magazine or something else that is relaxing and simple.

During the exam itself, read the entire exam from beginning to end, and find out how much time should be allotted to each individual problem. Once writing the exam, should more time be taken for a problem, it should be abandoned, in order to begin another problem. If there is time at the end, the unfinished problem can always be returned to and completed.

Read the instructions very carefully - twice - so that unpleasant surprises won't follow during or after the exam has ended.

When writing the exam, pretend that the situation is actually simply the completion of homework within a library, or at home. This will assist in forming a relaxed atmosphere, and will allow the brain extra focus for the complex thinking function.

Begin the exam with all of the questions with which the most confidence is felt. This will build the confidence level regarding the entire exam and will begin a quality momentum. This will also create encouragement for trying the problems where uncertainty resides.

Going with the "gut instinct" is always the way to go when solving a problem. Second guessing should be avoided at all costs. Have confidence in the ability to do well.

For essay questions, create an outline in advance that will keep the mind organized and make certain that all of the points are remembered. For multiple choice, read every answer, even if the correct one has been spotted - a better one may exist.

Continue at a pace that is reasonable and not rushed, in order to be able to work carefully. Provide enough time to go over the answers at the end, to check for small errors that can be corrected.

Should a feeling of panic begin, breathe deeply, and think of the feeling of the body releasing sand through its pores. Visualize a calm, peaceful place, and include all of the sights, sounds and sensations of this image. Continue the deep breathing, and take a few minutes to continue this with closed eyes. When all is well again, return to the test.

If a "blanking" occurs for a certain question, skip it and move on to the next question. There will be time to return to the other question later. Get everything done that can be done, first, to guarantee all the grades that can be compiled, and to build all of the confidence possible. Then return to the weaker questions to build the marks from there.

Remember, one's own reality can be created, so as long as the belief is there, success will follow. And remember: anxiety can happen later, right now, there's an exam to be written!

After the examination is complete, whether there is a feeling for a good grade or a bad grade, don't dwell on the exam, and be certain to follow through on the reward that was promised...and enjoy it! Don't dwell on any mistakes that have been made, as there is nothing that can be done at this point anyway.

Additionally, don't begin to study for the next test right away. Do something relaxing for a while, and let the mind relax and prepare itself to begin absorbing information again.

From the results of the exam - both the grade and the entire experience, be certain to learn from what has gone on. Perfect studying habits and work some more on confidence in order to make the next examination experience even better than the last one.

Learn to avoid places where openings occurred for laziness, procrastination and day dreaming.

Use the time between this exam and the next one to better learn to relax, even learning to relax on cue, so that any anxiety can be controlled during the next exam. Learn how to relax the body. Slouch in your chair if that helps. Tighten and then relax all of the different muscle groups, one group at a time, beginning with the feet and then working all the way up to the neck and face. This will ultimately relax the muscles more than they were to begin with. Learn how to breathe deeply and comfortably, and focus on this breathing going in and out as a relaxing thought. With every exhale, repeat the word "relax."

As common as test anxiety is, it is very possible to overcome it. Make yourself one of the test-takers who overcome this frustrating hindrance.

Special Report: Retaking the Test: What Are Your Chances at Improving Your Score?

After going through the experience of taking a major test, many test takers feel that once is enough. The test usually comes during a period of transition in the test taker's life, and taking the test is only one of a series of important events. With so many distractions and conflicting recommendations, it may be difficult for a test taker to rationally determine whether or not he should retake the test after viewing his scores.

The importance of the test usually only adds to the burden of the retake decision. However, don't be swayed by emotion. There a few simple questions that you can ask yourself to guide you as you try to determine whether a retake would improve your score:

1. What went wrong? Why wasn't your score what you expected?

Can you point to a single factor or problem that you feel caused the low score? Were you sick on test day? Was there an emotional upheaval in your life that caused a distraction? Were you late for the test or not able to use the full time allotment? If you can point to any of these specific, individual problems, then a retake should definitely be considered.

2. Is there enough time to improve?

Many problems that may show up in your score report may take a lot of time for improvement. A deficiency in a particular math skill may require weeks or months of tutoring and studying to improve. If you have enough time to improve an identified weakness, then a retake should definitely be considered.

3. How will additional scores be used? Will a score average, highest score, or most recent score be used?

Different test scores may be handled completely differently. If you've taken the test multiple times, sometimes your highest score is used, sometimes your average score is computed and used, and sometimes your most recent score is used. Make sure you understand what method will be used to evaluate your scores, and use that to help you determine whether a retake should be considered.

4. Are my practice test scores significantly higher than my actual test score?

If you have taken a lot of practice tests and are consistently scoring at a much higher level than your actual test score, then you should consider a retake. However, if you've taken five practice tests and only one of your scores was higher than your actual test score, or if your practice test scores were only slightly higher than your actual test score, then it is unlikely that you will significantly increase your score.

5. Do I need perfect scores or will I be able to live with this score? Will this score still allow me to follow my dreams?

What kind of score is acceptable to you? Is your current score "good enough?" Do you have to have a certain score in order to pursue the future of your dreams? If you won't be happy with your current score, and there's no way that you could live with it, then you should consider a retake. However, don't get your hopes up. If you are looking for significant improvement, that may or may not be possible. But if you won't be happy otherwise, it is at least worth the effort.

Remember that there are other considerations. To achieve your dream, it is likely that your grades may also be taken into account. A great test score is usually not the only thing necessary to succeed. Make sure that you aren't overemphasizing the importance of a high test score.

Furthermore, a retake does not always result in a higher score. Some test takers will score lower on a retake, rather than higher. One study shows that one-fourth of test takers will achieve a significant improvement in test score, while one-sixth of test takers will actually show a decrease. While this shows that most test takers will improve, the majority will only improve their scores a little and a retake may not be worth the test taker's effort.

Finally, if a test is taken only once and is considered in the added context of good grades on the part of a test taker, the person reviewing the grades and scores may be tempted to assume that the test taker just had a bad day while taking the test, and may discount the low test score in favor of the high grades. But if the test is retaken and the scores are approximately the same, then the validity of the low scores are only confirmed. Therefore, a retake could actually hurt a test taker by definitely bracketing a test taker's score ability to a limited range.

Special Report: Additional Bonus Material

Due to our efforts to try to keep this book to a manageable length, we've created a link that will give you access to all of your additional bonus material.

Please visit http://www.mometrix.com/bonus948/ccrnpediatric to access the information.